LORD I'M NOT DONE YET

A Believer's Guide to Accepting, Living, and Dying with Cancer

by

Phyllis Lomax Singh

Phyllis Lomax Singh

DISCLAIMER

This publication contains the opinions and ideas of the author. It is intended to provide helpful and informative material on the subject addressed within the publication. It is sold with the understanding that the author and or publisher are not engaged in rendering medical, health, or any other kind of professional services in the book. The reader should consult his or her medical, health, or other competent professional before adopting any of the suggestions in this book or drawing inferences from it.

The author and publisher specifically disclaim all responsibility for any liability, loss, or risk, personal or otherwise, incurred as a consequence, directly or indirectly, of the use and application of any of the contents of this book. Copyright 2014 by Phyllis Lomax Singh. All rights reserved, including the right to reproduce this book or portions thereof in any form whatsoever. For information address contact at: PhyllisLomaxSingh.com

LORD I'M NOT DONE YET
A Believer's Guide to Accepting, Living, and Dying with Cancer

Copyright © 2014 Phyllis Lomax Singh
All rights reserved.
ISBN: 1500854069
ISBN-13: 978-1500854065

DEDICATION

This book is dedicated to my family members who lived and died giving all they had to survive the battle of cancer.

***

Admit it, "Lord, I'm not done yet."

Live it, "Lord, I'm not done yet."

Shout it, "Lord, I'm not done yet."

***

ACKNOWLEDGMENTS

A special thank you to: my children Tammy, Jason, and Joshua for being my absolute reason for living; my best friend Sarav for giving me so much encouragement and support; my go-to doc Francois Theberge, MD for pushing me in the right direction when I doubted myself most during the writing of this book; and Peter Fotis Kapnistos, my editor who has the patience of a Saint.

CONTENTS

	INTRODUCTION	1
1	THE DIAGNOSIS OF CANCER - DON'T BE BULLIED	5
2	SECOND OPINION	9
3	TREATMENT OPTIONS WESTERN STYLE	12
4	EAST MEETS WEST	15
5	INFLAMMATORY PROCESS AND CANCER	17
6	ANGIOGENESIS	20
7	TOXIC CHEMICALS – MY HERITAGE	24
8	THE HEALTH OF THE MATTER	36
9	MAINTAINING GOOD NUTRITION	44
10	LOW ENERGY LEVELS	56
11	ACCEPT THE INEVITABLE AND SURRENDER	58
12	HOLISTIC HEALING APPROACH	61
13	BE POSITIVE AND ENCOURAGING TO SELF	66
14	DEPRESSION	72
15	PUSHING AWAY	76
16	THE DYING FAMILY	80
17	REGRETS	87
18	MENDING FENCES	91

19	LETTERS	94
20	FAITH AND MY DECISION TO FOREGO TREATMENT	101
21	MY NEAR DEATH EXPERIENCE	109
22	LAYING ON OF HANDS	113
23	COMPLIMENTARY AND ALTERNATIVE CHOICES	117
24	COPING WITH THE SIDE EFFECTS OF TREATMENT	125
25	MEDITATION	134
26	FAITH AND SPIRITUALITY	137
27	WHEN ENOUGH IS ENOUGH	140
28	FOOD FOR THOUGHT - MY FINAL WORDS	153
29	INVITE PHYLLIS TO SPEAK TO YOUR GROUP	158
30	REFERENCE PAGE	160
31	SHE IS OUR MOTHER	162
	ALPHABETICAL INDEX	164

Phyllis Lomax Singh

INTRODUCTION

More than one million people in the United States get cancer each year. Whether you have cancer or someone you love has cancer the information within this book is intended to educate, enlighten, and give you faith for a positive journey.

When a diagnosis of cancer is received it is like someone punches you hard in the middle of your belly. After a sharp intake of breath you can't breathe. The wind has been knocked out and you are drowning in the shock of the diagnosis. Your mind immediately numbs. The first thing you think is, "Am I going to die?" You may even say it out loud.

If you remember that day, stop reading for a moment and take a deep breath. I know you are reliving the painful memory of the news of cancer. I remember that day over and over as I reflect on the many ways I have heard the message delivered in my life time. Cancer has been, and is, my family's evil misfortune. My personal journey is the "why that makes me cry" and the reason I have written this book. I have been told whatever makes you cry within your soul is your pain, passion, love, regret, and reason for living.

We, you and I, are embarking on a journey to wellness. You can do this. I am here to guide you through your journey and to share with you ways to cope with the diagnosis of cancer, educate and enlighten you on ways to heal and nourish your body, mind, and spirit, discuss holistic alternatives to traditional Western Medicinal treatments, and to encourage you to live your life your way.

One thing to remember, life will never be the same. A diagnosis of cancer, regardless the type or severity of its progression, is a life changing, mind altering state of concern filled with fear and doubt. You can recruit family members, friends, cancer survivors, clergy, and physicians to help you sift through the mountains of information you will undoubtedly receive about your cancer diagnosis which may help you feel more confident as you choose your treatment path, but, you and only you can take control.

If there is only one thought you carry from this book, I pray it is knowing the difference between hope and faith. Hope is a feeling of expectation and desire for a certain thing to happen, whereas, faith is a complete trust or confidence in someone or something.

I can honestly admit I used the word hope in my vocabulary for many years. I was dependent upon hopefulness in my life. I even used hope when I prayed, "Lord, I hope to receive your blessings today. I hope you hear my prayer. I need blessings and hope you shower me with the blessings I need." Then I realized hope was a feeling, a desire within my heart, something I wanted to happen.

I changed my way of thinking when I realized I had wasted so much time hoping. I now have faith, faith and confidence. I am confident because I trust my choices and take credence in my walk through life and I want you to have the same.

Faith will help you cope with the days ahead and will aid in your decision making capabilities and it will help to:

- Reduce your stress, anxiety, and depression levels

- Improve your point of view
- Build confidence as you experience changes in your body
- Strengthen your drive and the will to live
- Provide a sense of inner peace within you
- Instill a satisfaction – You have lived your life your way

Phyllis Lomax Singh

THE DIAGNOSIS OF CANCER - DON'T BE BULLIED

Learning you have cancer is a difficult experience and after receiving the diagnosis, you may feel anxious, afraid, and even overwhelmed. You may wonder how you can cope during the days ahead. Planning your immediate future is very important for you and your loved ones. Obtain as much information as possible about your diagnosis.

Cancer by definition is a malignant growth or tumor resulting from an abnormal division of cells. Without control it invades other parts of the body through the blood and lymph systems and tends to destroy normal tissue. There are more than 100 different types of cancer and they are named for the organ from which they originate.

Cancer can also be grouped by systems:
- Carcinoma: a cancer that begins in the skin or in tissues that line or cover internal organs.
- Sarcoma: a cancer that begins in bone, cartilage, fat, muscle, blood vessels, or other connective or supportive tissue.
- Leukemia: a cancer that starts in blood-forming tissue such as the bone marrow and causes large numbers of abnormal blood cells to be produced and enter the blood.

- Lymphoma and myeloma: a cancer that begins in the cells of the immune system.
- Central nervous system cancers: a cancer that begins in the tissues of the brain and spinal cord.

You may have many physicians involved in your care and they may not have the same mindset for your treatment options. In addition to the doctors, you will have input from family and friends regarding how you should treat your disease. It is amazing how many armchair doctors are out there just waiting to give you their opinions. Do not allow anyone to "bully" you.

Remember, you and only you have control over your treatment. You have the right to make a decision based on information you are given. Do not let anyone rush you into a hasty decision. Taking time to decide may save your life! Let me repeat that – taking time to decide may save your life! Now, what do I mean by that?

One week will not make a difference in most cases and you need time to digest what you have been told, time to investigate your healing options, plan your recovery, share your love with family members, make necessary arrangements for your financial obligations, and decide who will manage your medical care as power of attorney in the event you become incapacitated.

Rushing into treatment and surgery does not allow anyone time to accept a diagnosis, understand what the diagnosis will mean as far as lifestyle changes, or have the information necessary for proper healing. Making hasty decisions adds a heavy burden of stress, anxiety, and fear, which affects the healing process in a negative way. The only reason to rush into surgery is when it is an absolute life and death need.

Unfortunately many doctors rush to decisions because their income depends on it. Insurance companies require diagnosis and plans of care for reimbursement. Without this the physician does not get paid. Offering alternatives to chemotherapy and radiation does not generate a large amount of revenue. Radiation and chemotherapy generates a great deal of income for the physicians involved with its administration. Statistically the success of these treatments are not worthy of the high cost related to the administration of the treatments. The quality of life is even less desirable with the conventional treatment of chemotherapy and radiation in that they destroy healthy cells along with the cancer cells and deplete energy necessary for the healing process. Any decline in mortality rates since the early 1990s is more than likely related to improved testing and early detection.

You may wonder what caused your cancer. The truth of the matter is you may never know the causative agent. It is said we all have cancer cells within our bodies but not everyone has active cancer cells. Cancer is caused by any chemical capable of altering human DNA and can be found in and around our environment, in the air, in our food sources, and even in our water. Other sources capable of modifying DNA are, genetically modified organisms (GMOs,) tobacco, air pollution, fluoridated water, pesticides and herbicides on produce, chlorine, and other contaminates found in our water just to name a few.

This is why it is of great importance to maintain a clean safe environment as well as consuming healthy foods in order to maintain good health. Natural lit spaces with clean air, nutritious food and water, and supportive social activities, free of toxins, promote good health, wellness, and healing. We can thrive if we have these conditions to live in and we have the tools to create this in our environment by making good choices for ourselves and our families.

There are Naturopathic physicians offering holistic choices for treating cancer but they are few and far between. Holistic cancer treatments are rarely placed in clinical trials because they are natural options and offer no side effects or dangers in administration. There is no loss of hair or burned skin and no damage to good cells along with the cancer cells. As a Certified Holistic Health Coach and a Registered Nurse, I coach cancer patients on holistic healing alternatives. I do not prescribe and am not a physician. I work with my clients in a way for them to make decisions regarding their healthcare through information for alternative modalities and a way for them to control their destiny without the damaging effects of radiation and chemotherapy.

I was blessed in making a choice to survive without radiation and chemotherapy. I attribute my good fortune to changes in lifestyle, an internal determination to disallow the disease process to ravage my body, and a deep faith in God to see me through the process.

SECOND OPINION

We have already determined receiving a diagnosis of cancer is a life changing event. Whether it is you or a loved one the news can be devastating. You may be experiencing many different emotions right now including feeling overwhelmed with all of the decisions that need to be made. All physicians, even though they are trained in the same specialty, do not treat illness in the same fashion. There are many routes to follow in treating an illness and curing a patient of a disease process. Second opinions can add additional treatment options for a specific type and stage of cancer, or it can confirm a treatment approach suggested by another physician.

Whether seeking opinions of an allopathic or holistic physician, it is important to understand the methods by which each treats specific illnesses and why. So, it is important to be armed with a list of identical questions for each physician in order to get an accurate representation of necessary treatment. If you ask different questions you do not get a second opinion – you get responses for treatment related to your questions which can in effect illicit different responses.

Seeking a second opinion allows you and your loved ones to be more informed about available treatment options. Learning as much as you can about your cancer and treatment plan can help you feel more in control of your path to a potential cure. A second opinion can give you peace of mind and help you feel more confident in choosing the right treatment plan for your disease process. Some specialty hospitals have treatments that are not available at general medical facilities. Seeking a second opinion from a specialty system like Cancer Centers of America where experts are committed to bringing the latest technologies and advanced treatment to patients sooner can be beneficial in the long run. They are supportive with therapies to reduce side effects, boost energy levels and keep patients as strong as possible during treatment. They have dedicated teams of doctors and other clinicians who will take time to understand your unique diagnosis and needs. They work together to develop cancer treatment plans including Integrative approaches to be used along with accepted Western healing concepts.

Have been told, "There is No Hope." I am here to tell you "THERE IS ALWAYS HOPE!" If your doctor says your cancer is untreatable, another doctor may be prepared to treat the cancer aggressively with surgery or chemotherapy, another may treat it with a combination of therapies, and you may choose to do as I did and treat yourself solely with diet, lifestyle changes, and a deep commitment to faith in God for your healing. Remember, don't be bullied! It is your life and death on the line not the doctors! You have nothing to lose and everything to gain by getting a second opinion and even a third.

Talk to your doctor about assembling a multidisciplinary team. It is important for success. The team can include but is not limited to:
- Surgical, medical, radiation, and naturopathic oncologists
- Registered Dietitian
- Certified Holistic Health Coach
- Nurse Care Manager
- Social Worker

I suggest you take a family member with you to your health care appointments. Two sets of ears hear more information when the information you are receiving is shocking. Write down questions and concerns beforehand and take them with you. Maintain a journal and make entries with each visit as well as additional questions you may have along your journey, and document any problems you may need addressed on future visits.

Get the facts using the same set of questions for all physicians:

- What type of cancer do I have?
- Where is the cancer located?
- Has it spread?
- What stage is the cancer and what does it mean?
- What other tests or procedures do I need?
- What is my prognosis?
- What treatment options are available?
- What is your treatment recommendation and why?
- What are the percentages of success of these treatments?
- What are my alternatives to radiation and chemotherapy?
- How will the treatment benefit me?
- What can I expect during treatment?
- What side effects can I expect?
- What has been your experience with this type of cancer and treatment options?
- What quality of life can I expect with your choice of treatment?
- Who else will be involved in my care?
- Who will administer the treatments suggested?
- Who will coordinate the Team?

TREATMENT OPTIONS WESTERN STYLE

Conventional treatment in the Western hemisphere generally begins with radiation or chemotherapy depending on the type, location, and aggressiveness of the tumor or a decision to have or not have surgery to remove a tumor or mass. If you have had tests, and the result of these tests have confirmed a diagnosis of cancer, you will need to slow down and concentrate on the choices ahead. Some physicians steamroll patients into scheduling surgery as soon as possible. Sadly most patients do not question their doctor about other options and there are many alternatives available!

Many times tumors or an abnormal growth of cells is found during a surgical procedure. Whether a tumor is benign (cancer free,) or malignant (cancerous,) the patient does not have the opportunity to make a decision regarding the path of treatment because they are under anesthesia at the time the discovery is made. The surgeon makes decisions based on his experience and expertise. The surgeon is entitled by the surgical consent form signed by the patient prior to surgery giving the surgeon sole rights to all decisions involved in the process of the surgery. Surgery, in itself, is considered a localized treatment.

Once a diagnosis of cancer has been confirmed a referral to an oncologist is usually made. An oncologist is a physician specializing in treatment of cancer and they will determine the course of treatment specific to a cancer diagnosis. In most instances the oncologist will suggest radiation therapy or chemotherapy or a combination of both.

Radiation is used to kill cancer cells. Special equipment sends high doses of radiation directly to the cancer cells or tumor and this process destroys and keeps the cells from growing. Radiation, no matter how carefully directed, can also affect normal cells near the tumor. Radiation can cause severe burns, organ, and skin damage which can be extremely painful. Radiation is also considered a localized treatment.

Chemotherapy differs from surgery and radiation in that it is used as a systemic treatment. Chemotherapy drugs travel throughout the body to reach cancer cells no matter where they are located. Oncologists determine which drugs are best suited for each patient. This decision is based on the type of cancer, stage of cancer, the patient's age, documented medical problems, and medications the patient takes on a regular basis. It comes with a high price. Like radiation, chemo is given to kill cancer cells. It also damages normal cells. The toxicity of the drugs can cause a multitude of severe side effects including:

- Damaged bone marrow/blood cells: causing neutropenia or anemia
- Damaged cells of hair follicles: causing baldness
- Damaged cells lining the digestive tract: causing nausea and vomiting
- Damaged cells in the reproductive tract: causing sexual dysfunction in men
- Damaged cells in the reproductive system: causing sterility in women

The last option most physicians have is to tell a patient, "You have no options." More than once I have heard a doctor tell a patient, "You need to get your affairs in order." Unfortunately compassion is not everyone's virtue. Truly the best thing any oncologist can say is, "I have reached the limits of my capacity to heal your cancer. If you wish to explore other alternatives, I can guide you."

This is one thing I wish they could teach in medical schools around the world. Life is not over until the heart stops beating. I know doctors are aware once the heart stops the death of cells follow – but to give a patient a death sentence while they still have an opportunity to reverse their condition in my opinion is not acceptable. All patients should be encouraged to make lifestyle changes to effectively change the living environment in which the disease process strives to an environment whereby the cancer cells are choked out and obliterated. Integrative nutrition is now being added to many medical school curriculums as it is a proven method of treating inflammatory disease processes through the use of nutrition and herbal supplements.

EAST MEETS WEST

I spent years in the belief Western medicine is the only medicine. My scope of practice revolved around what I was taught and what was used in the areas of medicine I worked in. However as I matured, became educated, and opened my mind to Integrative treatments I came to realize Integrative Medicine has very effective alternative treatment modalities for end of life and cancer care among other illnesses. They are relatively pain free, and do not damage healthy functioning cells within the body. Integrative medicine is a combined approach that takes complementary, alternative, and conventional medicine into consideration. It's the point at which East meets West for wellness and is called CAM therapies.

CAM therapies take a different approach. Most are founded in A*yurveda* and Indian medicine - from the Eastern hemisphere. They rely on herbs and "natural" substances, including whole food, as-well-as a nurturing of the mind and body to achieve health and wellness through meditation and exercise.

Complementary and Alternative Medicine has six categories:
- Diet based: Foods known to maintain good health and in a diagnosis of cancer they are known to aid anti-angiogenesis by retarding growth and killing off cancer cells.

- Biologically based: herbal supplements, vitamins, proteins, botanicals, pro-biotics and other organic approaches. 80% of all cancer chemotherapeutic agents are botanicals in origin.
- Energy Medicine based: electromagnetic forces which work to identify a body's own energy field called "chi." These therapies include acupuncture, reiki, Qi gong, and homeopathy.
- Manipulative and Body based: such as chiropractic, osteopathic, reflexology, water therapy, and therapeutic massage - specifically therapies that rely on manipulation of structures and systems of the body to heal symptoms and medical problems.
- Mind-Body Medicine: focuses on interactions between the brain, behavior, and physical health, such as meditation, yoga, biofeedback, tai chi, and spirituality and healing touch by laying on of hands and prayer. Mental health and physical health - are intertwined, and this type of approach is being used more and more for pain control, cancer management, and is being explored to learn more about its immunity capabilities.
- Whole Medical Systems: are filled with holistic alternatives for treatment and have names like naturopathy, homeopathy, traditional Chinese medicine, and Ayurvedic medicine.

INFLAMMATORY PROCESS AND CANCER

When investigating inflammatory processes and cancer, I realized the importance of the relationship of one to the other. When a person has an inflammatory process in their body it adds a major risk of cancer development, and, when a person has cancer, they have an active inflammatory process brewing within their body. A specific diet should be followed by anyone with an inflammatory illness as well as one with cancer because it is the best alternative for creating a positive healing atmosphere through the intake of specific foods providing nourishment for healthy cells and specific foods to target destruction of cancer cells.

Not all health problems are avoidable, but, you have more control over your health than you may think. Research shows a large percentage of cancer-related deaths are directly linked to lifestyle choices such as smoking, drinking, a lack of exercise, and an unhealthy diet. What you eat—and don't eat—has a powerful effect on your health. Without knowing it, you may be eating many foods that fuel inflammation and cancer, while neglecting the powerful foods and nutrients that can protect you. If you change your diet and behaviors, you can minimize your disease and possibly even stop cancer in its tracks.

A chronic inflammatory disease is a medical condition which is characterized by an ongoing inflammatory process. Many diseases fall into this category. Many inflammatory processes are regarded as familial and tend to run in families even if not considered a hereditary form of cancer.

Inflammatory disease processes develop when the immune system has an inappropriate response to something it has been exposed to and develops into an autoimmune response confusing the body's response mechanism. The inflammatory process becomes persistent and requires treatment.

Chronic inflammation can cause damage to the body, and it can lead to serious problems depending on where it is located. Regardless the primary location of an inflammatory process in the body – it becomes systemic in nature and affects the entire body. The most common reactions to inflammatory processes are fatigue, lack of mental clarity, poor digestion, and pain.

Some examples of chronic inflammatory processes are: Cancer, celiac disease, lupus, chronic obstructive pulmonary disease, (COPD,) irritable bowel syndrome, (IBS,) atherosclerosis, arthritis, psoriasis, and a plethora of other conditions related to the immune system including but not limited to multiple sclerosis, fibromyalgia, and chronic fatigue syndrome.

Chronic inflammatory disease processes can cause great suffering. They require constant attention to the symptoms which may fluctuate with severity. Many times these disorders can lead to total disability. Close attention must be paid to diet and diet therapies. By controlling what you eat and how you eat the inflammatory process can be controlled and even completely eradicated.

Important tips for avoiding inflammatory processes:
- No fried foods.
- No white sugar.

- Reduce intake of red meat: totally eliminate if possible.
- Use meat as a flavoring or a side, not as an entrée.
- Keep all meat to a minimum.
- Avoid processed products made from animal scraps like hotdogs and deli meats.
- When eating pork, poultry, and fish buy organic, grass fed when possible.
- Add beans and other plant-based protein sources to your meals.

Organic whole foods are essential to healing and restoring body to normal health. Eat a selection of organic raw fruits and vegetables daily. Steam and bake food rather than grilling. Remember, charred food has been reported as cancerous.

Dr Andrew Weil, MD, director of the Center for Integrative Medicine of the College of Medicine at the University of Arizona suggests "high temperature grilling (and broiling) of foods that contain fat and protein (meat and poultry, especially) produces carcinogenic compounds called heterocyclic amines (HAs) that can raise the risk of colorectal cancer in those with a genetic predisposition to the disease and may increase the risk of other cancers." http://www.drweil.com/drw/u/id/QAA400186

ANGIOGENESIS

A diagnosis of cancer is one of the most dreaded situations someone can face. There is massive ongoing research to find a cure, but, we must realize lifetime mortality rates for most cancers have not really improved much in the last 50 years. Only prevention has made a significant dent in the rate of certain cancers. It seems the only improvement in cancer care has been earlier detection and more aggressive treatment.

Cancer generally appears as an inflammatory process somewhere in the body. So it makes perfect sense for the body to react. In most cases a healing process called angiogenesis occurs. The body responds to the intruder or injured area by sending a healing mesh of cells to the area to create greater vascularity. In other words the body builds more blood vessels for healing and nourishing the injured area. This process is how our bodies heal lacerations, puncture wounds. skin tears, and surgical wounds to name a few. Inadvertently the new mesh highway of angiogenesis feeds cancer cells instead of defending the body against its attack.

A basic holistic anti-cancer regime includes:
- Detoxification
- Intestinal and nutritional strengthening
- Building a stronger immune system
- Consuming a diet rich in anti-cancer/anti-angiogenic foods

These therapies address the underlying causes of cancer that are usually ignored by conventional medicine. There are other areas of life addressed holistically and we will talk about them later.

Are there currently angiogenesis inhibitors being used to treat cancer? Yes, but it is not my purpose to promote chemotherapeutic medications. I am here to discuss holistic approaches and natural options to healing the body of cancer.

Dr William Li, head of the Angiogenesis Foundation, a non-profit organization involved in cancer research, has devoted much of his life to the effects of anti-angiogenesis and food. He presents a new way to think about treating cancer and other diseases: anti-angiogenesis, preventing the growth of blood vessels that feed a tumor. The crucial first and best step: Eating cancer-fighting foods that cut off the supply lines and beat cancer at its own game. Watch and listen to his explanation in this video online: https://www.ted.com/talks/william_li

The Angiogenesis Foundation

Founded in 1994, the Angiogenesis Foundation is the world's first 501(c)(3) nonprofit organization dedicated to conquering disease using a new approach based on angiogenesis, known as the growth of new capillary blood vessels in the body. They have identified angiogenesis as the "common denominator" in society's most feared diseases. Their focus on this underlying process of many different diseases makes their approach as a medical organization unique. The Foundation is the recognized, expert voice, and champion of this new field of medicine.

Based in Cambridge, Massachusetts, the Angiogenesis Foundation's goal is to help people lead healthier, longer lives by restoring balance to blood vessel growth. Through research, education, and advocacy — with patients, physicians, researchers, industry, payers, and government — they enable patients to gain access to safe and effective treatments coming from the angiogenesis field for cancer, blinding diseases, wounds, and many other serious diseases.

As a scientific organization, the Angiogenesis Foundation is independent of any individual, institution, or commercial entity. They are committed to helping people around the world benefit from the full promise of angiogenesis-based medicine, and to make life-, limb-, and vision-saving treatments available to everyone in need.

Dr Li sites the following foods as anti-angiogenic:

- green tea
- strawberries
- blackberries
- raspberries
- blueberries
- oranges
- grapefruit
- lemons
- apples
- pineapple
- cherries

red grapes
red wine
bok choy
kale
soy beans
ginseng
maitake mushrooms
licorice
turmeric
nutmeg
artichokes

lavender
pumpkin
sea cucumbers
tuna
parsley
garlic
tomato
olive oil
grape seed oil
dark chocolate

Holistically, cancer is approached in a way to provide what the body needs to heal itself. Dietary changes can affect the way angiogenesis occurs. Foods specific to anti-angiogenesis can slow and even halt the progress of cancer.

For further information http://www.eattobeat.org/

Phyllis Lomax Singh

TOXIC CHEMICALS – MY HERITAGE

In widening my Holistic studies and to better serve my clients, I completed an Environmental Medicine course at the University of Arizona Center for Integrative Medicine. It was an Integrative approach to raise awareness about diseases that may well be related to environmental toxins. Needless to say, I was blown away with the information I received in this course. Although I was aware of many hazards we encounter in our daily lives, I was not prepared to hear of the large proportion of toxic chemicals we are exposed to without our knowledge mainly because we just don't think about it. It has prompted me to be even more diligent than ever! Toxic chemicals are in the air, on the land, in the water, and many times hidden within the workplace. They can be found in most over the counter cleaning supplies, as well as within compounds used to make food containers, and even in baby diapers.

It is important to maintain a clean safe environment as well as consuming an intake of a healthy diet free of genetically modified organisms which are found in pesticides and fertilizers. Natural lit spaces with clean air, nutritious food and water, and supportive social activities, promote good health, wellness, and healing. We can thrive if we have these conditions to live in and use the tools available in our community to create this in our environment by making good choices for ourselves and our families.

The communities we live in are many times dictated by where we were born, where our occupation leads us, and where we are most comfortable living. Be it rural, urban, or city dwelling, it is our personal responsibility to look into the community in which we have chosen to live and make sure we are dwelling in a healthy environment.

Ask yourself this: Have I chosen a safe environment in which to live? Are there toxins being released into the air, land, or water in my community? The next time you take a leisurely drive, look around; make yourself aware of your environment. Think about the directions the wind blows. Are there manufacturing plants nearby? If so, what chemicals do they use and are they emitted into the air via smoke stacks, or sewer via open drains? The next time you take a walk look at the path as you walk. Is there trash thrown about rotting and seeping into the ground? Are there containers stacked on an empty lot? Are there rodents lurking around dumpsters behind grocery stores? This is just a little food for thought to help you become aware of your environment.

My Heritage

I was born and raised in a community where steel mills, tire manufacturers, and automobile plants populated the outskirts of the city. The direction in which the wind blew on any given day was the determining factor of the number of people receiving the heavy laden air containing the greatest amount of toxins. I was aware of the orange clouds moving across the sky and knew by the acrid smell of the air which steel mill was at full production. I was not aware of the hazards in the air we were breathing nor the toxic effects on our community through the soil and waterways.

The sides of homes in the area bore the orange stains of the steel mill's fall out. I could tell when the automobile plant was in full swing because the air smelled like hot rubber from the wiring harness lines. My mother worked those harness lines and came home smelling like rubber each day. Even after a bath she wreaked of the smell of rubber at times.

On the property of each of the steel mills were ponds of stagnant water covered with a heavy rusty orange film. These ponds overflowed when it rained and drained into ditches and a river nearby. The orange trail could be seen as the water rushed forward in the river to where it drained into the next waterway. The ponds near the tire manufacturing company and car plants were stagnant as well and when overflowed they ran into the same creeks and rivers as the steel mills. Since their branches split and ran through our county it created an unseen toxic waste land. The only fishes able to survive the sludge were carp.

Some of the communities near the steel mills and car plants did not have city water. Most homes had wells for water and septic tanks for waste. I remember the acrid taste of the water. Some wells were extremely salty from high concentrations of iron and I never had to add salt to food when I cooked with the water from those wells. A little further north the water from the wells smelled like rotten eggs when it ran out of the pipes into the sinks. I now know it was more than likely hydrogen sulfide leaching into the wells from bacteria using decaying plants, rocks, or soil as their energy source.

I often wonder what we were exposed to with all those chemicals leaching into our water, soil, and air! The sad thing is – it continues today. Those same ponds remain in my hometown fed by new commercial companies still dumping their end product into those same ponds that over flow into the same river.

I am an only child with a fairly large extended family. Well, I used to have a fairly large extended family. My mother had ten siblings and my father five, for a total of 15 of which 12 lived to adulthood. Eleven married bringing the total of aunts and uncles to 23. My mother died from breast cancer and my father from brain cancer. Of the 23 remaining siblings and their spouses, 13 died from cancers of the breast, prostate, lung, liver, brain, or blood as leukemia. Of the remaining ten, four are living with cancer, three died from other causes and three are living free of a diagnosis of cancer. Let me make it easier to grasp:

23 (aunts and uncles) + 2 (my parents) = 25 total
19 of 25 = 76% familial cancer rate in aunts/uncles/parents

An important note to this information: all but two of these family members worked at one of the automobile factories and lived in the community within three miles of the steel mills and plants spewing toxins into the environment.
To add to these incredible statistics: there were nine cousins raised in this community including myself; One male cousin died of a Glioma of the brain; his brother recently diagnosed with an active primary cancer; one female cousin living with active Acute Lymphocytic Leukemia; one female cousin in remission with Non Hodgkin's Lymphoma, and myself currently free of cancer. Four different sets of parents birthed us.

5 of 9 = 55.5 % familial cancer rate in cousins

I am a firm believer my family's predisposition to cancer is related to toxins in the air, land, and water supplies of the community in which we lived.

Before my mother was ever diagnosed with cancer she made a decision regarding my future. She told me I would never work in the automobile plant and coerced me into a nursing program. Her mind was not wrapped around the thought of toxic exposures because she was not aware of what was happening to her own body at the time. She was more concerned about the heavy labor of having to stand at a conveyer belt eight hours a day wrapping tape around wires on the harness line. Back then we did not argue with our parents we did what we were told. She had no way of knowing I would spend more than eight hours a day in my occupation standing, bending, and lifting. I do not regret her (our) choices for me. I was meant to be a caregiver and a caregiver I am.

How to reduce Toxic Chemicals in the living environment

Toxic chemicals can find their way onto your shoes as you go about your daily lives. You have no idea where toxic chemicals reside in your miles of walking outside your environment. It is important to evaluate your environment carefully.

- Take off your shoes immediately upon entering the house.
- Leave shoes in a place for easy access near the door.
- Wear in-house shoes or slippers when in the house.
- If you have babies or toddlers remember they crawl around where everyone walks and even suck on things they find on the floor!
- Mop and run sweeper often
- Go green when you clean. Purchase green products for your home http://www.greenhome.com/
- Stay informed and order the go green newsletter service http://www2.epa.gov/newsroom/gogreen

Water

As mentioned in the chapter, The Health of the Matter, water is pretty clean as it comes from our water providers, but, you can add a level of safety by adding a carbon filter for purification if you chose to. This will remove lead and chlorine and any bacteria remaining. If you live in an older home – let the water run for a few minutes before filling your glass or pot for cooking. Old homes are known to have lead in their pipes.

Never use water from the tap if it is discolored. Make sure your family knows not to use the tap water. Collect a sample of the water in a clean glass jar and seal it with a lid. Place it in an airtight bag and label it with date and time collected and notify your water provider as soon as possible. They may ask for a sample for testing and may even have you store it in the refrigerator so additional bacterial growth does not occur. Most times they will come and test the water so they have a fresh sample. Many times they will know why your water is discolored especially if there is a water main breaks in your area.

Food

Food brought into your home should not have any genetically modified organisms known as GMOs used in the process of raising, processing, or storing of food products.

Tips about food:
- Buy raw organic when possible.
- Never eat charred or burnt meat, both are carcinogens.
- Do not use containers known to contain BPA.

Air

Air inside our homes is generally more contaminated than outside air because of lack of circulation in the home. Off gassing can occur from carpet, drapes, and materials used in construction of furniture. Dust accumulation affects asthmatics and those with seasonal allergies.

Tips about air:
- Open windows and allow air to move through the house when weather permits.
- Purchase an air purifier if you can afford one.
- Use hepa filters when vacuuming.
- Maintain house plants. They provide oxygen and can remove toxic chemicals from the air.

In living and bedroom areas, dust and dander accumulation can cause flu-like symptoms and respiratory problems. Go Green by using non-toxic cleaning products to keep your home safe and save the environment. Natural cleaning agents are readily available in most stores.

Dry Cleaning

Dry cleaning and moth balls emit off-gas perchlorethelyne, a recognized carcinogen. Tips related to dry cleanable clothing:
- Hand-wash items that are dry-clean only.
- Use an eco-friendly dry cleaning or wet cleaning service.
- If you must dry clean – keep your dry cleaned clothing in a different place – not in your clothes closet.

- Take your clothes out of the plastic bags and air them for at least four hours before wearing them.
- Avoid products that contain synthetic fragrances by choosing fragrance free cleaning products or those made with essential oils. This simple change helps protect your health, your family's health, and other people within your environment. The FDA documented fragrances are responsible for 30 percent of all allergic reactions.

Pesticides

Stop using pesticides and use effective alternatives that are non-toxic to the environment. There are many home recipes out there that are safe and non-toxic. Another environmental culprit is chemical lawn treatments.
- Let your lawn go green — literally!
- Switch to environmentally-friendly alternatives instead.

Plastics

Get Rid of Toxic Plastics they have the potential to leach carcinogens and other dangerous chemicals that can affect your endocrine system. Some research has shown that BPA can seep into food or beverages from containers that are made with BPA. Exposure to Bisphenol A, (BPA,) is found in polycarbonate plastics and epoxy resins used in the manufacturing process of containers used to store food and beverages. It is also used to coat the inside of tin cans in which our food is stored and can be found on all grocery shelves in the world.
- Use BPA Free Plastics.
- Switch to glass storage containers.

Microwave

While a "microwave-safe" or "microwavable" label on plastic containers only means that they shouldn't melt, crack or fall apart when used in the microwave, the label is no guarantee that containers don't leach chemicals into foods when heated. The USDA also warns on its website against microwaving in single-use containers not intended for that purpose, such as takeout platters and margarine tubs. According to the FDA, microwave-safe plastic wrap should be placed loosely over food so that the steam can escape and should not directly touch your food.

For safety's sake, it's best not to heat foods in plastic and use ovenproof glass or ceramic containers with covers. Never use plastic storage bags, grocery bags, newspapers or aluminum foil in the microwave. Here are a few suggestions you can follow to reduce plastics and toxic exposure in your home:

- Avoid single-use disposable packaging.
- Buy food in glass or metal containers.
- Avoid heating food in plastic containers.
- Bring your own containers to salad bars, yogurt shops, etc., anywhere you'll be served in plastic.
- Avoid plastic cutlery and dinnerware, especially when cooking or heating food; use stainless steel or wooden utensils and look for recycled paper products.
- Use wood instead of plastic cutting boards and spray your wooden board with a mist of vinegar, then with a mix of hydrogen peroxide, to kill bacteria.
- When purchasing cling-wrapped food from the supermarket or deli, slice off a thin layer where the food came into contact with the plastic and store the rest in a

- glass or ceramic container, or non-PVC cling wrap. (see Shopping Suggestions)
- You can also write a letter to manufacturers of food and drink packaged in plastics, indicating your concern about plastics—especially if their packaging is #3, #6 and #7. Tell them you are actively seeking products packaged in safe, reusable glass, metal and recycled paper. Ask manufacturers for a mailing address by calling their toll-free question/comment line, usually listed on the back of the product; alternatively you can find their mailing address on their website

Glass, ceramic, and stoneware are the safest options when it comes to food packaging and storage because they do not leach any questionable chemicals when in contact with food. Unlike plastic recycling, which can produce toxic chemicals, glass recycling is more environmentally friendly. I buy organic in glass jars when I can find it – it is much safer. I also heat more in the oven after finding out all of this information about microwaving.

- Opt for glass or cardboard packaging; store your food in glass or ceramic containers.
- Seek cardboard to-go packing.
- Rinse all canned food thoroughly.
- Switch to stainless steel drinking bottles and non-plastic microwaveable containers.
- NEVER microwave food in plastic.

Antibacterial Soaps

Antibacterial soaps can cause big problems. It kills all bacteria, the bad and the good. It can create antibiotic resistance, meaning that certain bacteria can become immune to it over time. You can avoid these toxic problems by using only natural hand and dish by switching to a natural product.

Teflon Pans

Teflon Pans or non-stick pots and pans are great for non stick cooking but the chemicals used to create the lining of nonstick cookware can damage your liver or thyroid, or cause problems with your immune system. Choose iron, porcelain-coated, stainless steel, or glass pots and pans instead.

Personal Care Products

Everyone assumes their cosmetics and personal care products are safe to use. Don't be fooled by the expense of products the FDA doesn't even regulate them. You must be diligent in investigating products that contain dangerous ingredients like mercury, lead, formaldehyde, placenta, and animal byproducts.

Look for natural cosmetics and personal care products, especially those you use them on your children. Just a hint: most nail polishes and hardeners contain formaldehyde.

For lead and radon visit: epa.gov/radon/radontest.html.

Hazardous Waste

Treat cleaning supplies as hazardous waste. Hazardous waste is any product that is poisonous, toxic, flammable, or could mix with other chemicals and cause an explosion or dangerous reaction. Check with your disposal company for disposal rules and how to properly discard toxic cleaning supplies in your area. Many cities and towns have regular collection days or local collection sites that can take the toxic items and will dispose of them properly. Contact your local Department of Public Works for more options. Read the label: The CDC recommends checking with the manufacturers' instructions for disposal, which can sometimes be found on the label; if not, check with their website for more info.

THE HEALTH OF THE MATTER

Barring a genetic defect we are born healthy. Our body is strong and resilient in its construction. It is a magnificent engine of digestion, absorption, extraction, decomposition, energy production, and elimination of liquids and solids. It does all of this automatically without direction from our mind and it is geared to function in good health from our birth. Unfortunately, our bodies become sick or dysfunctional when we fail to provide the proper needs to keep it well functioning much like an automobile.

When anyone buys a new automobile it comes with a book providing data for upkeep and maintenance. If we fail to have the oil changed, air checked regularly in the tires, replace filters and mechanical parts at specific times geared toward age of the vehicle – it begins to break down. Our bodies do the same thing.

You may catch an airborne virus by breathing in the droplets from the air you breathe which has various ways of altering or destroying bodily function but you in effect may be responsible for causing a specific disease to plant itself within your body which can cause destruction, malfunction or lack of function, and even death by your negligence or by way of making bad choices.

Your body functions on a specific process. You nourish it by eating food and drinking liquids. It digests and absorbs what it needs and is capable of storing the excess of what our body uses to function, and it expels the remainder as waste as long as the body is healthy.

WATER

Hydration is extremely important to bodily function and maintenance. Should you drink filtered or bottled water? This is a matter of personal choice. I believe our water purification plants, on the whole, do their job. What causes contamination problems is related to the pipes through which the water is carried and whether there is a leaching of metal and chemicals from inside the pipes or a leaching from the outside through illegal dumping of toxic materials from manufacturer's or disposal of harmful chemicals through lack of knowledge of the harmful effects it can have on our environment and the water supply. If tap water was not safe the population on earth would be at zero.

I do not like the taste of water coming directly from the tap. I can smell and taste the chemicals in the water. I fill containers free of PBA and let them sit on the counter which I use for cooking and the making of hot drinks, and I refrigerate water for at least 24 hours to use as drinking water. I like my drinking water iced cold.

Having said most tap water is safe to drink, I admit to having used a filtration system at one time or another in the past. I have used bottled water at times but I make sure the plastic is BPA free. Be sure to pay close attention to the information on BPA in the chapter Toxic Chemicals. The body uses water:

- to replace what the body loses in sweat, urine, evacuation of bowels, and breathing
- to maintain normal body temperature
- to lubricate and cushion joints
- to provide protection for the brain and spinal cord
- to aid in removal of waste through urination, perspiration, and bowel movements

You need more water:
- When you live in a hotter climate
- When the temperature is hotter outside
- When there is an increase in physical activity
- When you sweat from overheating
- When you are running a fever
- When you have vomiting or diarrhea
- When you are detoxing
- To increase energy
- To relieve fatigue
- When you are on a high fiber diet

"The amount of water in the human body ranges from 40-60%.... Body composition varies according to age, gender, weight and fat content according to my trusted nursing textbook from Mosby's Inc., in Chapter 7 and 20, Body Systems/Electrolyte Balance 2010, 2007, 2003."

Do you know what happens when your body stores an excess of water? It causes an accumulation of fluid in the tissues causing swelling and compromises circulation and often times raises blood pressure. Swelling occurs mainly in the feet, ankles, and legs, but, it can also accumulate in the trunk of the body and in internal organs and their spaces, which can cause major problems in normal functioning of the body. Paying attention to water intake is as important as the intake of food.

FAT

Now let's talk about fat. There are conflicting opinions about eating fat. It is essential for proper body function. Fat makes it possible for other nutrients to be absorbed and utilized by the body, and when too much fat is accumulated we become overweight or obese.

Forms of fat:
- Oils are any fat which exists in liquid form at room temperature. Oils are also any substance that does not mix with water.
- Fats are mainly those which are solid at room temperature.
- Lipids are all types of fats, regardless of whether they are liquid or solid.
- Animal fats are butter, lard, cream, fat found in meats.
- Vegetable fats are made from a variety of vegetables including but not limited to; olives, peanuts, flax seed, corn, sunflowers, grape seed, coconut, etc.

Understanding fats can be a nightmare. For the most part of my existence this issue has been the most confusing in relationship to my diet because of the tug of war about fats and whether we need them or not! Let's break it down and make it easier to understand. Fats are needed to build nerve tissue and hormones, cushion and protect our internal organs, provide fuel because it is a concentrated source of energy, and is stored in your body for future use. If you don't use the fat you consume it stays in your body and this is where the problems begin.

There are three main types of fat unsaturated, saturated, and trans fat. Unsaturated fats are usually found in plant foods and fish. Unsaturated fat is good for the body and the heart. Examples include Tuna, Salmon, Avocados, and Vegetable oils - Olive, Peanut, Canola, flax seed, corn, sunflowers, grape seed, and coconut, etc.

Saturated fats are found in meat and other animal products, such as butter, shortening, lard, cheese, and milk (except skim or nonfat), palm and coconut oils. Saturated fat is generally solid at room temperature. It's also the fat found on red meat and poultry. Saturated fat should be used in moderation. ***Eating too much saturated fat can raise blood cholesterol levels and increase the risk of heart disease.

Trans fats are found in margarine, processed snack foods, baked items, and most commercially fried foods. They are also known as hydrogenated unsaturated fats. These fats should be avoided entirely. Eating trans fats can raise blood cholesterol levels and increase the risk of cardiovascular disease.

A few tips on how to reduce the amount of fat in your diet:
- Replace commercial bagged snacks with organic fresh or dried fruits and vegetables
- Poach, steam, grill, or bake your food. If you grill food do not char - charring has been linked to cancer
- Use almond, rice, soy, or low fat milks and replace fats with vegetable oils or limited amounts of butter
- Remove processed food and beef from your diet. If you must eat beef – eat lean grass fed beef in limited amounts

Healthy fats:
- Extra virgin olive oil
- Nuts
- Seeds
- Avocados

CARBOHYDRATES

Carbohydrates are often blamed for weight gain. But carbohydrates aren't all bad. They have many health benefits and are necessary in your diet. Your body needs carbohydrates to function well. Some carbohydrates are better for you than are others.

Carbohydrates are found in many foods and beverages. Most carbohydrates are naturally occurring in plant-based foods, such as grains. Food manufacturers also add carbohydrates to processed foods in the form of starch or added sugar. This is why processed foods should be limited or completely avoided to prevent inflammatory disease and cancer.

Common sources of naturally occurring carbohydrates include:
- Fruits
- Vegetables
- Milk
- Nuts
- Grains
- Seeds
- Legumes

There are three main types of carbohydrates sugar, starch, and fiber. Sugar is the simplest form of carbohydrates. Sugar occurs naturally in fruits, vegetables, milk and milk products. Sugars include fruit sugar (fructose), table sugar (sucrose) and milk sugar (lactose).

Starch is a complex carbohydrate. A carbohydrate whereby many sugars are bonded together. Starch occurs naturally in vegetables, grains, and cooked dry beans and peas. Fiber also is a complex carbohydrate. Fiber occurs naturally in fruits, vegetables, whole grains, and cooked dry beans and peas. Fiber is a healthy carbohydrate and helps the gut stay healthy.

Carbohydrates are used by the body as its main fuel source. Sugars and starches are broken down into simple sugars during digestion and are absorbed into the bloodstream where they are known as blood sugar (blood glucose). Glucose enters the cells with the help of insulin. Glucose is used for energy and fuels all bodily activities. Excess glucose is stored in the liver, muscles and other cells for later use or is converted to fat.

Carbohydrates are an essential part of a healthy diet and should be chosen wisely:
- Emphasize fiber-rich fruits and vegetables. Choose a variety of whole fresh, frozen and canned fruits and vegetables without added sugar.
- Choose whole grains. Whole grains are the best source of fiber and other important nutrients, such as selenium, potassium and magnesium.
- Low-fat dairy products. Choosing low-fat versions will help limit calories and saturated fat.
- Beans and legumes. Legumes, peas, and lentils are the most versatile and nutritious foods available. They are low in fat; contain no cholesterol; and are high in folate, potassium, iron and magnesium. They also have beneficial fats and soluble and insoluble fiber. They are a good source of protein and are a healthy substitute for meat.

PROTEIN

Protein is broken down during digestion into amino acids that are used to build new proteins facilitating communication between the cells inside our bodies. Protein can also yield energy when there is a shortage of fats or carbohydrates. Protein is found in the following foods:
- High quality natural cheeses and yoghurt, omega-3 enriched eggs, skinless poultry and lean meats
- Legumes

- Tofu
- Eggs
- Nuts and seeds
- Milk and milk products
- Grains

MAINTAINING GOOD NUTRITION

After receiving a diagnosis of cancer, a patient's thoughts often turn to treatment options and prognosis. Many have had surgery, radiation therapy, and chemotherapy, or a combination of any of the three. Most of their questions and concerns are about how they will get through it. Nutrition is not likely to be on their list of immediate concerns but it should be.

Good nutrition is important for everyone. But what exactly does good nutrition do for a patient with cancer? Not only will cancer patients reap the benefits of being healthier and better able to withstand treatment but the right food can choke out active cancer cells.

Patients with different types of cancer will have different nutritional needs. Everyone needs nutritional screening initially and periodically throughout the healing process as problems occur with lack of appetite or inability to eat. Nutritional screening and specific courses of dietary supplementation are not a universal component of cancer care, but again, it should be! Evidence that diet can prevent cancer or the recurrence of cancer is mounting and has been well documented in recent years.

Eating a well-balanced diet and maintaining a good nutritional state can keep you strong and provide the nutrients your body needs to heal its self and recover. Better nutrition empowers the body to heal faster. Good nutrition can eliminate side effects of treatment, improve quality of life, and raise the chances of survival significantly.

By providing the right tools a cancer patient can experience feelings of empowerment as they take control of their nutritional health which can allow them to tolerate their treatment and improve their quality of life, which by all means is the most important part of cancer treatment.

Good nutrition provides:
- A store of nutrients to maintain and rebuild healthy tissue
- A decreased risk of infection
- An increase in strength and energy
- An improvement in immunity function
- An enhancement of your overall well-being

Symptoms present red flags regarding nutritional status when conventional cancer treatments cause side effects which make it difficult to stay nourished:
- Fatigue
- Loss of appetite
- Altered sense of taste/smell
- Nausea/vomiting
- Weight loss
- Mouth sores
- Difficulty swallowing
- Diarrhea/constipation
- Radiation burns
- Uncontrolled pain
- Anxiety
- Depression

Planned good nutrition can keep a person strong and provide the nourishment the body needs to heal itself. The stronger the body the faster it can heal. Cancer can affect the entire body and its function. It is important to monitor weight, fatigue, nausea, constipation, diarrhea, and anemia states.

- Monitor your weight closely to ensure you are maintaining a healthy weight.
- Take frequent rest breaks throughout the day and eat small, frequent meals every three hours of nutrient-dense foods to give you more energy.
- During periods of nausea maintain a low-fat, bland diet of cooler foods, and drink ginger or cardamom tea to settle the GI tract.
- Increase your fiber intake and drink fluids throughout the day to maintain hydration.
- Adding Psyllium flakes to drinks can aid smooth evacuation of bowels by adding much needed soft fiber to your diet especially if you are taking narcotic pain relievers.
- Iron supplements can be added at the discretion of your physician to increase red blood cell count.
- Organic Unsulfured Molasses can add much needed potassium without the problem of swallowing large pills.

It's important to address any nutritional problems as early as possible. A Registered Dietitian can provide a detailed nutritional assessment to evaluate nutrition status, identify micronutrient needs or inadequacies, and determine the most appropriate nutrition interventions. A Naturopathic Clinician can recommend appropriate vitamin and mineral supplementation. A Holistic Health Coach can assist in reviewing lifestyle changes needed to meet a healthy healing environment.

It is important to eat frequent small meals. This maintains a constant nutritional state within the cells. Eating every three hours incorporating a variety of fruits and vegetables with a healthy protein and a carbohydrate also keeps stomach from overfilling and triggering nausea. It is important to pay attention to your body:

- If you become constipated - increase fiber and water intake.
- If you notice an increase in gas limit carbonated beverages and gas forming vegetables.
- If you have mouth sores - avoid acidic drinks.

Experiment with your food. Try flavoring foods with seasonings and spices to improve the taste. If you can't eat solid foods - drink shakes and smoothies made with fresh or frozen fruits and vegetables. They are very tasty and nourishing. Additional protein and carbohydrate needs can be supplemented with many available OTC prepared nutritional drinks. Be selective and be sure to avoid drinks containing genetically modified ingredients which are harmful to the body.

Try to drink 8-10 glasses of water each day. Unsweetened juice, broths, smoothies or shakes are a great method of adding hydrating fluid to your body. If swallowing is difficult, suck on frozen fruit cubes or popsicles.

Keep mealtime interesting, vary the time, place, and surroundings. Make a tray and eat on the porch. Pack your lunch in a bag, grab a bottle of mineral water, and go to the park. Sit on a park bench and enjoy the peaceful surroundings. Make mealtime interesting. Find quiet, pleasant, and soothing atmospheres. Most of all find good company to share a meal with!

When investigating research regarding inflammatory processes and cancer, I realized the importance of the relationship of one to the other. When a person has an inflammatory process in their body it adds a major risk of cancer development, and when a person has cancer, they have an active inflammatory process brewing within their body. So this diet should be followed by persons with an inflammatory illness as well as one with cancer. Adding natural foods to a diet is known to retard cancer growth and reduce inflammation without causing harm to our bodies.

HEALTHY SWEETS NO SUGAR! Avoid white sugar - use small amount of date syrup to sweeten your food. Everyone has a need for sweets or a craving at times. The important thing is to eat healthy sweets when you need them and eat them sparingly. Healthy choices are unsweetened dried fruit, dark chocolate, and fruit sorbet. Dark chocolate provides polyphenols with antioxidant activity. Choose dark chocolate with at least 70% cocoa and have one ounce twice weekly as your treat. Chocolate forms flavanoids during the fermentation process and they are highly concentrated in dark chocolate and cocoa powder. Catechins and procyanidins may protect against cardiovascular disease and cancer.

TEA 2-4 cups daily. Healthy choices are white, green, Matcha, and oolong teas. Tea is rich in catechins and antioxidant compounds that reduce inflammation. Purchase high quality tea and learn how to properly brew it for maximum health benefits. Oolong tea has chemo preventive properties and is best used against cancer.

RED WINE is a matter of personal choice, 1-2 glasses per day. Healthy choices are Organic red wines. Red wine has high powerful antioxidants shown to have anti-cancer, anti-inflammatory, and heart-protecting effects.

HERBS AND SPICES are used in unlimited amounts of fresh or dried or powders. Healthy choices are turmeric, curry powder, ginger, garlic, onion, chili peppers, basil, cinnamon, rosemary, thyme, and cayenne.

Three ingredients one needs to consume daily in raw, cooked, or powdered form are onions, garlic, and turmeric. This is a must! Use herbs generously to season foods. Turmeric, garlic, and onions are powerful, natural, anti-inflammatory agents as well as anti-cancer agents. According to the American Institute for Cancer Research, garlic may lower your risk for colon cancer with compounds that block tumor formation and cancer cell growth in the colon.

PROTEIN SOURCES 1-2 servings a week which is one ounce of cheese, one 8 ounce serving of dairy, one egg, three ounces steamed or baked skinless organic chicken. High quality natural cheese and yoghurt, omega-3 enriched eggs, organic skinless poultry, and grass-fed lean meats. It is important to eliminate or reduce to a minimum your consumption of red meat. If you must eat red meat – be sure it is lean, grass fed beef and eat sparingly.

Try to eliminate animal foods. Much of what we derive from these foods actually increases inflammation, so, removing them from your diet will help reduce you inflammatory state. If you must eat red meat purchase lean cuts of grass-fed beef. When choosing poultry it is important to choose organic free range poultry and buy skinless variety. Use organic dairy products and keep them at a minimum. Buy omega-3 enriched eggs. These are made by hens consuming a flax meal enriched diet.

WHOLE SOY FOODS 1-2 servings daily 1/2 cup each. Healthy choices are tofu, tempeh, edamame, soy nuts, and soy milk. Soy foods contain isoflavones that have antioxidant activity and are anti-cancer agents. Soy may lower the risk for breast and prostate cancers. One caution: Some studies have noted a reduction in fertility and sex drive with soy consumption.

FISH AND SEAFOOD 1 serving daily equal to 4 ounces of fish or seafood. Healthy choices include wild Alaskan salmon, herring, sardines, and black cod. These fish are rich in omega-3 fats which are strong anti-inflammatory agents. Eating fish produced on farms as opposed to wild-caught fish add concern related to antibiotics, pesticides and other chemicals used in raising farmed fish may have harmful effects to people who eat the fish, so it is important to buy fish caught in the wild.

HEALTHY FATS 5-7 servings daily equal to 1 teaspoon of oil, 2 walnuts, 1 tablespoon of flaxseed, and 1 ounce of avocado. Healthy choices for cooking are extra virgin olive oil. Healthy fats include nuts, avocados, and flaxseed. Grind flaxseed prior eating, or buy ground instead of whole, to better absorb the nutrients. Healthy fats are rich in monosatunsaturated and omega-3 fats. EVOO is rich in polyphenols with antioxidant properties. The protective benefits of nuts most likely come from antioxidant compounds like folic acid and magnesium, according to a research review in the *American Journal of Clinical Nutrition*. Consumption of flaxseed is known to increase levels of endostatin a known cancer inhibitor.

GRAINS 3-5 servings daily equal to ½ cup cooked grains. Healthy choices are brown rice, basamati rice, buckwheat, barley, quinoa, and steel-cut oats. Whole grains digest slowly reducing frequency of blood sugar spikes which promote inflammation. Compared with refined grains (like white bread and regular pasta), whole grains have much more fiber, which may protect against colorectal cancers because it helps move food through your digestive system faster.

PASTA 2 servings per week equal to ½ cup cooked pasta (al dente.) Healthy choices are organic pasta, rice noodles. Pasta cooked al dente has a lower glycemic index than fully cooked pasta. Low-glycemic-load carbohydrates should be the bulk of your carbohydrate intake to help minimize spikes in blood glucose levels.

BEANS AND LEGUMES 1-2 servings daily equal to ½ cup cooked beans or legumes. Healthy choices are black, chick peas, fava, lentils, dahl, pinto, cannellini, and kidney beans. Beans are rich in folic acid, magnesium, potassium, and soluble fiber. They are a low–glycemic-load food. Eat them well cooked either whole or pureed into spreads like humus. Read How to prepare lentils and beans.

Beans are comparable to meat when it comes to calories. Our diets tend to be seriously skimpy when it comes to fiber. One cup of cooked beans (or two-thirds of a can) provides about 12 grams of fiber - nearly half the recommended daily dose of 21 to 25 grams per day for adult women (30 to 38 grams for adult men). Beans are pretty much the perfect food. Refer to Preparing legumes for proper cooking technique.

Note: Having meatless meals can slash your risk for cancer, so consider eating more beans such as black, pinto, lima and kidney as well as other legumes like lentils and black-eyed peas. Postmenopausal women whose diets contain lots of beans have lower rates of invasive breast cancer.

VEGETABLES ORGANIC 4-5 servings daily equal to unlimited mixed salad greens, 1 cup vegetables, cooked, raw, or juiced. Healthy choices are all leafy greens – spinach, collards, kale, and Swiss chard, cruciferous vegetables – broccoli, cabbage, Brussels sprouts, cauliflower, Bok choy, carrots, beets, onions, tomatoes, and squash. Vegetables are rich in flavonoids and carotenoids with both antioxidant and anti-inflammatory properties. Eat a variety of colors for balance of nutrients. Eat raw and cooked. Eat organic vegetables. Brussels sprouts, cauliflower, cabbage and broccoli pack sulfur-containing compounds that may inhibit the growth of cancer cells. Studies have linked them to lower rates of lung, liver, colon, breast and endometrial cancers. Dark green leafy vegetables are loaded with folate, a B vitamin that helps repair damaged DNA that's vulnerable to cancer. Some studies suggest it may guard against GI cancers in particular – and possibly breast cancer too.

FRUITS-ORGANIC 3-4 servings daily equaling 1 medium fruit, ½ cup chopped fruit, ¼ cup dried fruit - no sugar added. Healthy choices are Raspberries, blueberries, strawberries, black berries, peaches, apples, nectarines, oranges, grapefruit, grapes, plums, pomegranates, pears – all lower in glycemic index than tropical fruits. Fruits are rich in flavonoids and carotenoids with antioxidant and anti-inflammatory properties. Eat a wide range of colors.

Choose fruit that is in season, fresh, or frozen. Buy organic when possible. If using frozen be sure it is with no sugar added. Berries contain antioxidants that reduce and repair the kind of damage to cells that can lead to cancer. When they're not in season, choose frozen berries since they're typically just as healthy as fresh. Red and purple grapes contain the same disease-fighting compound found in wine – resveratrol – which has been shown to slow the growth of cancer cells and block tumor formation in the liver, stomach and breast. Lycopene, the pigment that gives grapes their color, also boasts cancer-fighting properties.

WATER

Water intake is very important. Take your body weight and divide it in half. This is the number of ounces of water your body requires daily. For example: If you are 180 pounds – you would need 90 ounces of water daily. This is nearly three quarts of water. Fill a container with the number of ounces you are required and place it in the refrigerator. Drink from this container during the day – making sure you drink all of it. You can have other beverages as well but you must drink the proper amount of water. It is preferable to drink filtered or bottles spring water.

Note: If your physician has limited your fluid intake for medical reasons – it is imperative you follow his directions. Again fill a container with amount of fluid your are allowed. Remove water from that container to prepare your coffee, tea, or other beverage and plain water for drinking. Water for you is not extra. Your total fluids are being monitored for your health. It is very important to adhere to this practice. Water is vital for bodily function. It keeps its temperature normal, lubricates and cushions your joints, protects your spinal cord and other sensitive tissues, gets rid of wastes through urination, perspiration, and evacuation of stool.

Note: If you have had a problem with constipation or hard stools, adding fiber can help elimination. Psyllium flakes (one teaspoon) added to a beverage is tasteless, adds a nice consistency to a chilled drink, and helps to keep waste soft and moving.

Another habit to get into is – upon waking drink a quart of warm water with ½ teaspoon of sea salt. Generally bowels will move within 30 minutes. This will help regulate those who have no bowel regulation due to unhealthy lifestyles.

Dr Andrew Weil suggests the best way to obtain all of your daily vitamins, minerals, and micronutrients is by eating a diet high in fresh foods with an abundance of fruits and vegetables. In addition, supplement your diet with the following antioxident cocktail:

- Vitamin C, 200 milligrams a day.
- Vitamin E, 400 IU of natural mixed tocopherols (d-alpha-tocopherol with other tocopherols, or, better, a minimum of 80 milligrams of natural mixed tocopherols and tocotrienols).
- Selenium, 200 micrograms of an organic (yeast-bound) form.
- Mixed carotenoids, 10,000-15,000 IU daily.
- The antioxidants can be most conveniently taken as part of a daily multivitamin/multimineral supplement that also provides at least 400 micrograms of folic acid and 2,000 IU of vitamin D. It should contain no iron (unless you are a female and having regular menstrual periods) and no preformed vitamin A (retinol). Take these supplements with your largest meal.
- Women should take supplemental calcium, preferably as calcium citrate, 500-700 milligrams a day, depending on their dietary intake of this mineral. Men should avoid supplemental calcium.

Other Dietary Supplements

If you are not eating oily fish at least twice a week, take supplemental fish oil, in capsule or liquid form (two to three grams a day of a product containing both EPA and DHA). Look for molecularly distilled products certified to be free of heavy metals and other contaminants.

Talk to your doctor about going on low-dose aspirin therapy, one or two baby aspirins a day (81 or 162 milligrams).

If you are not regularly eating ginger and turmeric, consider taking these in supplemental form.

Add coenzyme Q10 (CoQ10) to your daily regimen: 60-100 milligrams of a soft gel form taken with your largest meal.

If you are prone to metabolic syndrome, take alpha-lipoic acid, 100 to 400 milligrams a day.

For further information on Dr Andrew Weil's dietary supplement suggestions visit http://www.drweil.com

LOW ENERGY LEVELS

Low energy levels not relieved by adequate sleep or relaxation techniques may be caused by poor nutrition. However, if you are constantly feeling drained, low energy levels may be a symptom of an underlying medical problem such as metabolic dysfunction, depression, anxiety, treatment modalities such as chemotherapy and radiation, or anemia.

If you have had a history of a chronic state of low energy it may be more difficult to correct. Possible causes for low energy can be caused by long-term illnesses that have gone untreated, such as anxiety, depression, or abnormal lab values caused by poor absorption in the gut due to poor dietary choices and eating habits and can worsen with an inflammatory disorder or cancer.
Low energy levels can slow the healing process and healing takes a great deal of energy, so you must provide the body with high levels of energy through good nutrition and a healthy state of mind. I believe mindset is as important to treatment for healing as food consumption and environment.

We have all experienced energy drains – a day when we have been so exhausted we can't find the initiative to even move from the sofa. It is suggested a walk around the block would help to increase energy. Although I agree, I have found when you are feeling horribly drained from an illness, distance walking is out of the question while a smaller effort to walk is a start. Do your best to walk inside your home. Open the windows and allow the outside to come in. When you feel up to it venture out into the yard or onto your porch for a short trek a few times a day. Breathe in the fresh air and allow the sunlight to grace your presence. Add a little distance each time until you can eventually take that walk around the block.

Take a power nap. I am a big fan of power naps. It seems when you are an older adult or experiencing an illness whether short lived or extended – power naps are a wonderful way to rejuvenate your energy stores.

Don't skip meals. Make sure you are consuming the calories and nutrients needed to heal your body and to replenish your stores.

Reduce stress. Stress drains the energy store more than any other activity because it affects the mental, physical, and emotional parts of our being. It is a rare person who can contain stress in one area over the other. When stress affects the mind with its racing thoughts it overflows into the body resulting in tensed muscles, and emotionally as mounting fear and concern.

Have a Power Snack. Have fresh fruit with some hard cheese or nuts. This is a quick pick me up for loss of energy. Enjoy a large glass of water with your snack. Many times we mistake hunger for thirst. So replenish both while you are at it!

And lastly or firstly, however you will have it - don't for get to worship God. Give God the glory for all He does for you daily. Give thanks and praise for your day. He has given you the breath of life and He will see you through this trial. Give your worries to God and He will fill you to overflowing with the energy you need.

ACCEPT THE INEVITABLE AND SURRENDER

It takes a lot of letting go of control to accept the inevitable. It is important to realize there are aspects of life beyond our personal control. The sun comes up every morning without fail: winds blow, birds sing, and sirens blare when an emergency arises. The only thing we have real control over is how we think; our actions, our speech, how we engage with others, and even what we allow others to know about us. Admitting our beliefs, conditionings, and methods of existence belong specifically to us and are not the underlying foundation for everyone else's beliefs, conditionings, and methods of existence is a major revelation.

The reality is that each and every one of us is experiencing life through a different set of existing influences; different vantage points, lifestyles, family relationships, financial statuses, faiths, and life dreams. Imagine that.

To accept and surrender is accepting, honoring, and respecting those differences. When you can appreciate others for their way of doing things even when it is different from your own method of doing things it will allow a peaceful atmosphere within your heart. So it is important to honor differences.

Don't try to change anyone. Allow them to do things their way. You may have opinions, give suggestions, and allow them to make the choice of whether to use the information or not. But, the decision of whether or not to act on your suggestions must rest within their personal choices. I say these things in order to ease into the subject of acceptance and surrendering to the diagnosis of cancer. I do not suggest you surrender as in "lie down and give up," but in the acceptance and understanding of your disease process and what it takes to reverse it. Accepting the inevitable is a must. Say it, "I have cancer." Accept it and plan a path to heal yourself. For without acceptance and surrender you cannot succeed in healing yourself. You will inadvertently place road blocks to your successful healing path.

You must accept you have no control as far as the diagnosis you have been given but you can however influence the outcome of your disease process by maintaining a supportive healthy fit lifestyle in order to reverse your cancer. How you approach cancer and receive its existence within your body will determine how well you are committed to reversing your illness. There is no assumed path for everyone to follow – your path to healing should incorporate your personal set of existing influences.

Practice harmony, balance, dis-ease, peace, and surrender. It is important to let go. When you are able to let go and accept your cancer - you will feel it in your being. Allow grace to consume your soul. Living in a state of surrender is the ultimate goal. Living in a state of surrender will determine the end result of your efforts. If you are not familiar with the term dis-ease, not to be confused with disease, it is a term used by holistic healing communities aligned with wellness. It infers we choose not to empower health issues by focusing on a specific ailment but to place emphasis on the natural state of "ease" being imbalanced or disrupted.

It is also important to nourish a rich and intimate inner dialogue with yourself, an ongoing conversation with that inner voice existing in the soul of your subconscious awareness. The ability to cure one's self may come as a big shock to many people but I firmly believe we have the internal power to heal ourselves by the grace of God.

Dr Kelly Turner, MD in her book, Radical Remissions stated, "Many of the patients had healed without undergoing Western medical treatment or, following its failure, they used other therapies to extend their survival" She went on to say there were 9 factors common to most of the patients:

- Made a radical change in their diets
- Took control of their health
- Followed their intuition
- Used herbs and supplements
- Released suppressed emotions
- Increased positive emotions
- Embraced social support
- Deepened their spiritual connection
- Had strong reasons for living.

Our bodies are a marvelous machine capable of correcting its problems if given the proper fuel and tools. There are many ways in which to empower yourself to heal your body from an affliction. It is important to believe in the healing process, know the steps to take for healing, and take them. Empowering the body to heal itself is easy when the proper steps are taken.

HOLISTIC HEALING APPROACH

A holistic healing approach is when a person chooses to treat imbalances within the conscious and unconscious parts of their body's existence which influences the outcome of their health. Most times physical health is a result of an imbalance in lifestyle brought on by poor dietary choices, stress, lack of exercise and rest, continued exposure to toxins in the environment, and/or the ignoring of an active inflammatory process within the body. Physical discomfort, lack of energy, and mood changes are generally the first signs of imbalance.

The difference between holistic the healing approach and western medical treatment is that the physical health may not be the main focus for the path of treatment. While pain and discomfort may be the main issue of a client, the source causing the imbalance must be found in order to change the outcome.

To give a few examples:

A person over exercises and feels pain in the muscles over used. Many folks immediately seek pain relief and call a doctor for pain pills and muscle relaxers when the best treatment is to massage the affected muscles gently and continue to exercise the muscle band slowly. When active exercise is resumed – it is important to not over tax the area – and to know when to stop. Pain medication is not always the best alternative.

Some people hate their jobs and awaken in the morning with their stomach in knots, feeling nauseated and dread about going to work. They have no immediate solution to being able to change their occupation or place of employment so how do they treat their symptoms?

Again most people seek prescription medications to decrease the amount of stomach acid created by their stress and something to relieve their nausea and pain and may even take medicines for anxiety but continue to assault their well being by making no change to relieve the stress of working in a place literally making them ill.

Holistically the stress of the job is addressed with an introduction of coping methods to be practiced to alleviate some of the triggers causing the physical problems. It is a proven fact stress is relieved by concentrated breathing exercises and stomach acid production is decrease by guided meditation. These simple exercises can be completed in the work place and can alleviate some of the associated symptoms until a person can change their place of employment or change their job entirely. Many times the job becomes tolerable because the client has learned to reduce the anxiety their workplace has caused through active dis-ease exercises.

Too many times we seek prescription drugs as a "curative method," and that is only a band-aid for the problem and many times creates new problems as well. Physical illness is a symptom of a greater imbalance within our bodies which require our immediate attention.

When is the last time your physician addressed or has he/she ever addressed the following with you when you were in the office for a specific medical issue other than symptoms related to your complaint?

- Career
- Education
- Finances
- Health
- Physical activities
- Home cooking
- Home environment
- Relationships
- Social life
- Joy
- Spirituality
- Creativity

Think about it. How long do you actually sit with your physician in their office discussing your medical complaint? The average physician spends seven to eight minutes interviewing, examining, and prescribing treatment for a patient illness or follow-up visit.

The majority of physicians do not know the number of children you may or may not have, what your common dietary choices are, or even, the occupation you have whereby a holistic practitioner will ask about all twelve aspects of your life and spend an hour discussing a plan of action which will work best with your lifestyle.

The holistic approach I follow is an ongoing practice to go far beyond the mind-body connection and to include spirituality and wholeness of life in the process. It involves physical healing, mental health and wellness, emotional well being, a spiritual connection, and a way to find and access the tools one needs to change imbalance to balance and well being. It is totally about a lifestyle approach to wellness.

When embracing a holistic approach to well being a person learns the importance of embracing the environment around them, maintaining healthy relationships, accepting changes necessary to find a healthy physical, mental, spiritual balance, and a way to heal the body from the inside out.

I am very fortunate to be empathetic in nature. God has blessed me with the ability to read beyond what a person shares verbally. I believe this has developed more deeply following my near death experience. As I matured and studied the gamut of modalities affecting my practice I incorporated a mix of western and eastern options.

Being empathetic allows me to assess deep emotions as well as a person's actions. Many illnesses run deep and are not portrayed because the client has subconsciously learned how to bury the emotions causing the health problem and don't even realize it themselves. As they have learned to hide the conflicting issue, I have learned to see it deep beneath the surface and address it making them able to feel at ease and not to feel as though they are alone as they learn to connect with the problem and find healing.

My empathetic nature allows me to know when to be compassionate, considerate, and even how to speak softly with someone versus using a normal or loud voice. Many times I am drawn to pray with a client and to lay hands on them in the name of God for healing.

I have read many articles about empathy and wish all medical workers had the ability to be empathetic. When reading the many traits associated with empathy I found I am deeply empathetic in nature and have been my entire life.

I have trouble accepting compliments and would rather point out someone else's tributes rather than my own. I am highly expressive in areas of emotional connections. I am an open book never afraid to share who I am with others. I am able to talk about my feelings and will cry with someone whether they are in my presence or in the distance. If they are experiencing pain whether it is physical or emotional I will connect with that pain. I tend to feel what is outside of my being rather than inside and ignore my own needs in lieu of others.

I am a problem solver, a thinker, and a studier of many things. Where there is a problem I know there is an answer and I will search and search for the answer. What is of no importance to another can be of utmost importance to me. I am non-violent and non-aggressive in nature and known as a peace maker. I am uncomfortable when there is disharmony in my space and will back away from the situation by finding a solution for the problem quickly. I seek to correct a misunderstanding quickly rather than to let it sit and fester.

I am sensitive to things I read, see, and witness and can be brought to tears when it affects my emotions. I tend to hate the telephone and lovingly embrace online communication with wide open arms. I love my personal time alone and enjoy my time with the Lord. All of these things have drawn me to who I am and to how I coach to find solutions for those in my practice.

BE POSITIVE AND ENCOURAGING TO SELF

Remember that which is nurtured blossoms and grows. Others can lavish encouragement and motivation for you to move in specific directions regarding your health situation, but, you must recognize that the force is inside you and the most effective motivation and encouragement must come from within you. You must be your biggest and most supportive cheer leader!

- Practice desirable behaviors and replace undesirable ones
- Reconnect with your reason to be positive
- Goal - Reverse cancer
- Heal myself - on my terms
- Create A Dream Board
- Make a poster with all of your goals and life dreams
- Post pictures of family members, places to visit, dreams to be fulfilled and place it where you can see it daily
- Add new dreams to your vision board as they arise
- Include goals for healthy fit lifestyle
- Write Down Your Accomplishments, place stars on those achieved

A person who learns to focus on the good they've already done in life will be much more inspired than someone who focuses on the things they lack.

Journaling

Journal daily – focus on the positive - no negatives here! Spend five minutes on the past, five minutes on the future, and five minutes on what you are grateful for. I totally believe in journaling as a healthy habit.

I used to journal faithfully. Sometimes I believe my writings kept me alive and moving forward in troubled times much like my gardening practice. Then someone I trusted destroyed the volumes of my poetry, my drawings, and my precious 16 life journals. With it my documented beliefs, philosophies, and private writings went up in smoke. To this day I can't bring myself to journal as a habit but I now post my musings, philosophies, and heartfelt opinions on the internet through social media posts, web pages, and blogs. So, in a way I am still journaling.

I must admit these postings are as cathartic as my journal writings were and many times more rewarding because they touch someone else's heart. They are no longer private. I do pine the loss of my journals more than the art because there were so many thoughts about the day to day joys my children brought me. The poetry can never be revisited except for those poems which were published and there have been several of those throughout the years. The pages destroyed were as much a part of me as life was, since I wrote about my struggles, accomplishments, and had expressed it in my drawings.

So I behoove you to keep your journals in a safe place so no one destroys your heartfelt writings. Maybe you want to share them with your family – especially the great memories you document. I don't consider myself a great artist by any means and I have never taken a painting class in my life but all the same I love what I create and it is a definite healthy de-stressor for me.

If you write a little each day and begin with the three things you are thankful for. It can be as simple as, I am thankful for the robin sitting on my fence. It can be one of the greatest experiences in your life if you allow it to be. It will slow your thoughts down and make you think.

After writing the three things you are thankful for write what you are feeling – the good, the bad, the beautiful, and the ugly. Write about things influencing the way you feel. You can even write down what you think you can do to improve a situation and go back weeks later and realize the problem is resolved.

You can journal about your life and make it a story of day to day living, like a diary of sorts, because that is what journaling is - a diary. Journaling is a way to encourage yourself in life by documenting your direction with points of departure and arrival – as though you are on a trip. You are on a trip after all – the trip of life.

You may actually discover you are someone totally different than you thought you were. It can make you aware of the things you live for and can give you clarity of thought. I used to doodle when I was thinking in between placing my pen to the paper and when I would revisit my journal pages I could remember the exact thoughts going through my mind as I drew cubes, faces, or flowers on the pages. Things like baseball bats and footballs always warmed my heart because I knew I was writing about my boys on those pages.

Journaling is all about personalization. You will uncover dreams and goals that you may never know existed. You may uncover additional reasons for living, for fighting, for healing the disease within you. It can give you a peace of mind and grow your spirituality and your faith and hope. By writing your feelings and thoughts on paper you open your soul to the universe and to God. It is different than prayer. I used to keep a notebook and instead of praying I would write letters to God. Now I use a "God Can" instead.

You can write about love, anger, jealousy, pride, resentment, faith, family, goals, achievements, encouragement, or anything in the world you want. It is your book, your journal, your heartfelt writings.

Time for "Me"

You must realize how important it is to make time for "me." I am sure throughout your life you have said things like "I wish there were more hours in a day," or "I don't have time for that." All of us have lived very busy lives and many times have ignored making time for ourselves because we are committed to doing things for others whether it is family, friends, or employers.

Most of us lead hectic lives but creating personal time is essential for good health. Finding as little as 20-30 minutes each day for "me" time can be a great health benefit. Taking time for ourselves assures a deeper sense of happiness, comfort, and even self esteem. That "me" time allows us the time to de-stress, unwind, and rejuvenate and greatly relieves dis-ease in an imbalanced body.

Never feel guilty over taking a little personal time it allows you the opportunity to come back with a positive attitude, a well rested feeling, and a less stressed mental state. If everyone around you is worthy of care and attention – so are you! If you're fighting an inflammatory disease or cancer you need it for healing. Without it you will feel frustrated, angry, weak, tired, overwhelmed and out of balance.

Remember, "Me" time is not selfish - it is part of self care:
- Look at the areas where you can rearrange your time to give you 20-30 minutes to call your own.

- Decide how you will spend your "Me" time to its best advantage.
- Put it on the calendar and keep the appointment.
- Evaluate things you waste time doing.
- If you are an online junkie like me – cut back. I spend hours researching and reading articles that many times are not my primary interest. I see hours wasted by people I work with as they constantly surf their phones for social media posts.
- Learn to say no when others infringe in your time. There is no sin in saying no to a request and don't be afraid to ask for help. There are others who can do the same thing you do and do not be afraid to ask.
- Commit 20-30 min of each day to "Me" time. I guarantee you will feel better!

Communication

Communication defined: to share or exchange information, news, or ideas...hmmm. I have seen patients and clients shut down after hearing the word cancer. It almost seems like they have had their vocal cords severed. In response to general conversation and questions they simply nod, annoyingly groan, loosely mumble, and even avoid making any noise at all. It happens as a defense mechanism. Silence somehow removes the problem because it is denied presence. Well this can't be right, can it?

Absolutely not! Shutting down only adds to the problem at hand. It is important to organize and clarify ideas in your mind and if you chose to not be in a specific conversation – say so. Being rude is hurtful to the receiver and this is not the time to create barricades that will need to be removed at a later time.

Be clear. Be sure what you're wishing to convey has a purpose in the conversation. Do not change the subject to suit your needs. Listen to the conversation. Others may have needs addressed as well and you can fulfill their need by being attentive to the subject at hand. Everything is not specifically about you, even though you may think nothing else is going on in the world around you. The disease of cancer is a family dis-ease. It is praying on everyone's thoughts, emotions and stress levels. As a family it must be addressed.

Stay on topic. Once you start speaking, make sure everything you're saying is truthful and adds to the conversation. Make sure you share your feelings and never, never, never be critical of others thoughts. Remember, they are also dealing with this overhanging cloud of cancer and are filled with doubts and concerns of your wellbeing as well as their own! Make every attempt to solve issues together. One person making the decision can leave discord in the family process and this is a time when the family unit must stay united.

Always thank those who have given you input during the communication of the subject at hand. Acknowledge their input as beneficial to your successful healing process. Even if you disagree tell them you will consider their suggestions. It will give them a satisfaction of being helpful even if you choose to not utilize their advice.

DEPRESSION

What does depression feel like? Depression never feels the same for everyone. It weighs down on a person's being and is experienced in different ways for different reasons. Some people may feel sad and without energy when depressed, while others may feel hopeless, alone, and unmotivated. Depression takes its toll as it depletes the minds ability to allow pleasure in life or actions. Most of the time a person just can't get moving and they don't want to.

Simple things become a challenge for many. They bulk at getting up in the morning and getting dressed. Sometimes the depression is so severe it affects one's appetite either by overeating or by not eating at all. Either way the body suffers the choice. As the time of depression is prolonged other illnesses can creep into the body and take seed causing a variety of new symptoms including fatigue, pain, lack of ability to concentrate as well as a host of others. Most people are affected at one time or another by depression either through personal experience or vicariously through a friend or family member but it is magnified tenfold when a person is suffering a terminal illness or cancer. Depression is a vicious cycle and it becomes easier to give into it than it is to fight it.

Depression manages to affect all people diagnosed with cancer or a terminal illness at one time or another and it occurs more frequently as the ill effects of chemotherapy and radiation leave a person with a feeling of being sick, lost, and alone.

Here are some of the symptoms of depression:
- Hopelessness
- Ongoing sadness
- Helplessness
- Loss of interest in activities or hobbies
- Decreased energy
- Increased fatigue
- Difficulty concentrating
- Insomnia or oversleeping
- Appetite and/or weight loss or overeating and weight gain
- Thoughts of death or suicide
- Restlessness and irritability
- Inability to deal with pain, treatments, family and friends
- Difficulty concentrating

There are many ways to deal with depression without the use of drugs. Depression requires a change in behavior. What happens inside the mind when a cycle of depression overshadows someone? It tends to get worse as a person takes on depressive behaviors such as staying inside, not getting dressed, or sleeping late to name a few. A person becomes complacent, unable to change the downward spiral of feelings, and it reinforces the lack of desire to go out, get dressed, or get up on time and fosters an even deeper depression.

Recently a dear friend of mine, Nancy, posted on social media how depressed and tired she was feeling following her most recent round of chemotherapy. She admitted it had left her exhausted and she was terribly embarrassed to be seen with her lack of hair. Immediately suggestions came to her post by loving and caring friends. Most of the posts were a resounding affirmation she should force herself to get up and move regardless how she felt about her appearance. As friends, everyone shared their feelings about her being an inspirational self empowered woman and no one was giving her a break or an excuse to give up.

A few days later I found myself laughing and crying at her next post. I was cheering and pumping the air with my up stretched arm for her pup and yelling, "You go Cami!" Although my friend was ranting and raving about how she was forced to get dressed and leave the house even though she had no desire or energy to do so, the dog was my hero! This was her post:

"Today was great. Does anyone want to adopt my rotten little dog? First, she tore two bags open and made a mess of the contents. Then she escaped and ran all over the neighborhood like a bat out of H***. She ran into the stinky creek behind our house and got wet. So I put her in her crate to think about her behavior, let her out and she acted like a maniac running all over the house. My grandson loved chasing her and she hated being chased, so she jumped up onto my CLEAN bedding, including the bedspread, which I just put back onto my bed 15 minutes ago after washing and drying it, which only took 3 hours. And in the excitement, she PEED on my bed! I am so upset right now about this; I could tear my hair out, if I had any.

On a more upbeat note, I did go outside this morning for about 15 minutes. I hate the heat and humidity, but it was good to go out. And I drove all over the neighborhood while my granddaughter chased the goof ball dog trying to catch her. So these are two things that got me out. I also made some no bake cookies for the grandkids. I am really trying to limit sugar, but I needed a cookie. Oh, my-gosh, I did not remember how sweet *those cookies are. I will be lucky if I get one down. But that's a good thing. I know when I stay away from sweets and chocolate, I really can do without them. Don't miss them or crave them, again, a good thing. Okay. Thanks for letting me rant. Now I must go wash my bedding all over AGAIN. Later!"*

Even today, I still feel like cheering for her pup. Cami was able to do for my friend what we as a collective could not do for her. Sometimes I am truly amazed how God can use animals to help us get out of our own way! I can see my friend in her frustration shaking her finger through the cage at the pup in one instant and hugging her to her heart in the next saying, "Thank you."

Depression is a state of mind directly linked to mood and thought processes. When a person thinks negative thoughts they begin to believe in the negativity, so it is important to replace the negative thoughts with healthier ways of thinking. Exercising the mind is an excellent way to do this. To believe in the healing process and to say it out loud is much more productive than thinking it.

Physical exercise, meditation, and breathing exercises help combat depression as well. It stimulates the body, its internal organs, and the mind. It increases circulation as well as the hormones used by the body to maintain its mental balance.

PUSHING AWAY

There are many cancer patients and those who are terminally ill who will immediately begin pushing others away following their diagnosis. Somehow they reason It will be easier when I die if I leave them now, I will protect them from the pain of my disease process if I stay away from them, or I will not let them see me struggle.

The reasons are endless but in reality the 'pushing away' is the most devastating. I am going to share my personal experience in hopes it will impact upon you the importance of why you should not push people away. Instead draw them to you, hold them close, and love them every moment you can!

My parents were divorced when I was a toddler. My father spent most of his life in prison and was never really in our lives. He never provided financial support to help with raising me. My mother worked at a local automobile plant from the time I was a small child. She provided total and complete care for me with the help of her eldest sister, Elsie. I can never remember her raising a single hand to me, or raising her voice for that matter, but, when she was upset with me she would become silent. Her silence was the harshest punishment she could have delivered to me as a child.

I craved communication. I was a latch-key kid from the age of four. I was expected to be responsible and act like an adult because there was no money for a baby sitter and I was told if I let anyone know I was alone the welfare people would carry me away. I learned the behavior and was left alone from five in the morning until five in the evening. My food was left in the refrigerator and on the table and somehow I managed to not burn down the small apartment in the project in which we lived. I share this specific information with you to allow you a glimpse into the pain I revisited when my mother pushed me away after she received her diagnosis of cancer.

My parents were both in the end stages of cancer when it was discovered. They were diagnosed within months of each other. My mother had end stage breast cancer forcing her into medical retirement. She lived with me. My father was diagnosed with end stage brain cancer while in prison and I was forced to assume care for his wellbeing when the prison system decided he was no longer a risk to society and was costing them too much money to provide end of life care for a comatose prisoner. I had to place him in an extended nursing facility due to his comatose state.

Struggling with the severity of what life had dealt me was enough, but, my mother in her great wisdom to protect me from her demise stopped communicating with me. Days passed and she would walk past me in the house and not utter a word. She would spend hours chatting on the phone with a young woman for whom she babysat prior to her cancer discovery. They would make plans to go shopping on the weekends and go out to dinner in the evenings. When I asked if I could take her out for her birthday I was informed she had made plans with her friend.

My mother was mobile until the last two months of her life at which time I became her total caregiver. I gave her loving care in silence all the time wondering what I had done to deserve the silent treatment as when I was a child. Four weeks before her death the young woman she had chosen over me came to visit my mother who was now bedfast. She sat at my mother's bedside laughing and sharing the latest news of her child's activities. I listened to their happy exchange and became angry. My mother shared no words with me other than to ask for her pain medicine or to have a massage on her painful back. I felt as though I would explode my heart ached so much with the pain of being shut out.

I barged into the room and shouted at my mother, "How dare you!" with tears streaming down my face. I could barely get the words out but I continued yelling, "I am your daughter! You have grandchildren who love you. I am taking care of you day and night, and you sit here with your friend laughing and listening to her stories about a child who is not your grandchild?" I fell to my knees at her bedside not caring about what her friend thought. I sobbing and asked, "What have I done to you that you hate me so much? You have grandchildren who aren't allowed to come inside this room, but, you share the pictures of a child you babysat as if she is all you love in this life!" There are tears in my eyes as I write this – it is as if it happened yesterday the pain in my heart is so great. It still festers every time it crops into my mind.

My mother reached for my hand and I jerked it back as if her touch would burn me as she said, "I don't hate you or my grandchildren. I love you." I shook my head no as she continued, "I thought it would be easier on you when I died if I kept a distance from you while I am sick." She was wrong. It only created a painful memory for me. I was jealous of her friend. I was hurt. I did not understand why she found the need to punish me. I was ashamed before God. I was ashamed for yelling at my mother. I was ashamed for not confronting her sooner in a way not to hurt her.

Through the years since her death this memory crops up without reason - my mother went into a coma three days after I yelled at her and died three weeks after the verbal exchange. I did apologize for my outburst and voiced my love to the woman who bore and raised me, but, the wound is still there, weeping for the time we lost when she made the decision to push me away! Lost moments, lost time, lost love, lost memories forever!

THE DYING FAMILY

When it comes to a diagnosis of cancer, it not only affects the person diagnosed with the illness, it also affects family and friends. I have always addressed a diagnosis of a terminal illness in a mind set of: the dying family. Having experienced cancer so many times in my own family, I have learned the complexity of feelings, emotions, and unplanned changes in lifestyle can be overwhelming. Learning to accept and understand the changes you will face and the way they relate to you will help your path to healing by fostering a healthy healing environment, nurturing mutually supportive relationships, and sharing love and compassion for each other as you address your disease head on.

Relationships spouses/partners

Cancer has a huge effect on married couples and long-term partnerships. Both partners will experience a plethora of emotions; sadness, anxiety, anger, and hopelessness. There may be major changes in relationships and in the way a household is reorganized to compensate for chores and/or family activities. For many partnerships facing the challenges of cancer together strengthens their relationship and commitment while others with a troublesome relationship prior to the diagnosis of cancer, drift apart with the stress of cancer and the problems it creates within an already tumultuous relationship, or, the relationship is maintained without support being given to either partner leaving a heavy burden of guilt if a partner dies from the disease.

Cancer affects each relationship individually in respect to family dynamics prior to the diagnosis. Cancer can change the roles of partners. Where one partner may become overbearing, overprotective and controlling, another may become withdrawn, distant, and quiet. Both of which can effect communication during the treatment phase, healing process, and many times the process of preparing for the loss by death.

Often spouses obsess about cure and fail to take the feelings or wishes of their partner into consideration when making decisions. It may help the non-cancer spouse cope with the illness but it adds a tremendous pressure to the cancer bearing partner. It is important to remain flexible and listen to each other's needs.

Adjusting to changes in roles does not come easily. A person who has always been the caregiver may have trouble adjusting to a more dependent role, while a person who has not been a caregiver may struggle to take charge and provide needed care.

These changes in relationship dynamics may even fall to other family members of the affected couple whereby children are drawn into major roles of giving or aiding in care by way of providing care for the cancer affected parent or by being given the responsibility of caring for siblings in the absence of parents.

Communication

It is important to talk with your spouse or partner and work together as best you can to make decisions about treatment, care giving, and other issues. Family dynamics is an integral part of the healing process. All changes affect each member of the family. A formulated team approach to the illness is essential. Everyone's emotional well being must be considered. Take time to sit and discuss the options available and take notes outlining the family plan. Make sure your wishes are heard! *Remember live your life your way!*

In most relationships there is an ongoing partnership of designated day-to-day duties. One may cook, run the sweeper, and carry out the garbage, where the other pays bills, buys groceries, and brings in the mail. Unfortunately these chores no matter how well divided pre-illness can become troublesome post diagnosis. A redirection of previously designated chores can alleviate feelings of frustration, exhaustion, and worry. Simple tasks can be delegated to even young children without overwhelming them with changes and yet give them a feeling of pride in helping the family.

Because physical and emotional needs change frequently as families cope with cancer, it is important for everyone to communicate their needs. All family members need reassurance that they are loved and included in the community of family. Open communication makes sure this message is heard resoundingly by all members of the family.

Effects of cancer on your relationships with friends and family members will vary depending on the communication and coping styles of each person. Everyone reacts differently to crisis situations and it is important to plan your strategy for communicating news and asking for support.

Family and Friends

Although it may be difficult for both partners, it is important to accept help from extended family members and friends. Don't be ashamed of asking for assistance. Give them the opportunity to help. Let your needs be known and allow them to love you by being there to help. It will also give them an opportunity to feel pride in an accomplishment of being there in your time of need.

Many families are torn apart over misunderstandings and choices made when there are disputes about aggressiveness of care versus comfort care for a dying family member. Everyone needs to understand how much hurt can result leaving things unsaid. For example - many times one sibling will want to continue aggressive treatment for a parent while another seeks to discontinue treatment and give comfort care. The reasons for their difference in opinion may come from an entirely different place. One may be thinking of the parents needs while the other may be feeling guilt over their relationship with the parent or lack of relationship and seek to remedy it through a feeling of doing all they can at the end of life to make up for a failed relationship. Disputes of this nature are rarely healed and are important to address head on to save the family unit following death.

Set goals

Cancer often changes future family plans. Working together to meet new, short-term goals can help families feel more connected. Things that seemed important before the cancer diagnosis may take a back seat to more pressing priorities; spending more time together; securing a healthy fit lifestyle; beating cancer, etc. Some goals may be put on the back burner and can be addressed at another time rather than abandoning them completely.

Who is in Charge of Relating News?

Be specific about your needs and try not to make assumptions about who will help and who will not. Prepare a list of things others can do for you and allow them to come into your daily life and help alleviate your responsibilities as you see fit. If they become a pest do not be afraid to redirect them by saying, "I need to rest for the next few days – let me call you when I feel up to a visit."

It has been my practice to ask patients and clients to appoint one person to call for updates. Not to mention it is exhausting to phone every family member after every test result or doctor's appointment. I feel this is a very important process to continue. Rely on this trusted individual to communicate with family members the information about test results and plans of care. It is important to choose someone who will relay your information without changing facts, someone who will treat your information with respect, and someone who faithfully informs other family members regarding your progress.

You may find family members and friends avoiding conversation. They may avoid talking with you because they don't know what to say. Others may simply avoid talking about cancer for fear it will upset you.

If there one thing I can reinforce with an absolute mind set is talk about your cancer process. When you feel like talking about your cancer, bring up the subject with your friends and family members, and let them know that it's okay for them to talk about it. Reassure them that you don't expect answers or wild plans for a cure but you only want them to listen and try to understand your feelings. It is also okay to tell people when you don't want to talk about your cancer as well. It is totally up to you whether to share or remain private in your daily thoughts.

Children

When it comes to your children it is important to realize your children have excellent hearing even when they appear to be playing. They will learn about your diagnosis from other adults instead of you. They need to hear about it from you. Second hand information can lead to an understanding the conversation is taboo and can prevent the child from going through the grieving process which is essential for their acceptance and understanding of the illness. Open and honest communication about cancer or any other illness in a way that is appropriate and adheres to your children's temperament and your family values is the best way to communicate about your terminal illness. It will strengthen your bonds and help your children deal with the experience in a positive way. Failing to include them can cause a lifetime of psychological issues including but not limited to anxiety, fear, doubt, love, and trust issues.

Very young children can sense that something is wrong and even they need honest information to help them cope. Keep in mind ages of your children and give them truthful and accurate information they can understand but facts which won't overwhelm them. Focus on things that will affect them directly, such as changes to their schedules or changes in your appearance, which might be more frightening if the changes are unexpected.

Expect changes in children's behavior as they adjust. Younger children may become overly clingy, impulsive, and needy. Older children or teenagers, on the other hand, may become angry, withdrawn, verbally expressive, and even challenging of their previous set boundaries in an effort to cope with your illness.

Normal daily schedules are important. Encourage them to ask questions and let them know it is okay to talk about their feelings and fears. Reassure your children that they will always be cared for and that you will always love them.

Spirituality

Terminal illness brings with it a struggle with questions about mortality, the meaning and purpose of life, and whether a greater power exists in the minds of those unfamiliar with faith and God. As a Believer, I accepted Christ as my Savior when I was eleven years old. I did not always lead an exemplary life and I made many mistakes in my journey thus far but one thing I am sure of: there is a God, He hears our prayers, knows our needs, and has a plan for us whether we agree with it or not.

If you are not practicing faith, please know you do not need an invitation to begin a conversation with God. It is never too late to introduce God into your life. Praying is simply talking to God. God knows your heart and is not concerned with your words as much as He is with the attitude of your heart.

It is important to be grateful for what you have been given in your life no matter how small it may seem at this moment. God deserves the glory for without God we would be nothing. Having faith in a Creator and believing your disease can be healed is essential to your progress.

Worshiping as a family can be tantamount in the ability of a family to deal with the disease process. It can comfort, give peace mind, and strengthen family ties.

REGRETS

Are you having regrets? Is there a little voice inside you secretly asking why, or, is there a booming voice inside you screaming? Regret has two paths of burden and emotion. Regret can be something you feel you have done wrong to someone or something; it can also be something you wish you had stepped in and done differently to change an outcome as you look back over your life.

One thing to understand, blame or guilt will not change the deep hurt you feel over regret. Many people feel regret without a life changing event, but, when it comes with a terminal illness it can be debilitating. It is important to deal with it even though it can cause great pain and deplete energy needed for healing as you go through the emotional process.

Review your regrets. Are there things you wish you had done and now feeling the time slipping away? These are things you may still be able to do:

- I wish I had not worked so hard and spent more time with my family.
- I wish I had kept in touch with my friends.
- I wish I had taken vacations.
- I wish I had saved more money.

Or, are your regrets about something you consciously chose to do and it in some way caused harm to someone or something? You may have made many decisions in your life which affected others.

Always tell someone how you feel, because opportunities are lost in the blink of an eye but regrets can last a lifetime...
Carson Kolhoff

I will share with you a deep regret one of my clients experienced and how it was handled. Right or wrong the pain of her actions runs deep. The pain is unending and is felt by her daughter and herself. It would take a book in itself to bring you to where she was when she made the decision to leave her young daughter in her grandmother's home in order to protect her from an abusive step-father.

My client's decision unknowingly scarred her daughter for life. Even though my client maintained a close physical presence in her daughter's life maintaining a loving non-abusive living environment for her, it left a negative impact on their relationship which may never be whole again. Even though she has apologized to her daughter many times the pain of her decision constantly weighs upon her heart.

Because my client allowed her work, personal life choices, and lack of financial ability to dictate her choices, her daughter painfully denied her visits to the grandchildren for ten years. She has not seen her daughter or her grand children for over five years following the severe sanction. She sends gifts and knows they are aware a grandmother exists but my client does not call her daughter's home for fear one of the children will answer and she will break her promise to her daughter.

She waits patiently for her daughter's weekly call on Saturday or Sunday where exchanges of words are made with no mention of an immediate solution in site. My client's biggest fear is she will die before she has the chance to see her grandchildren. She is resolved to accept her daughter's decision regardless the pain it causes in her heart. My client is more concerned about her daughter's welfare than her own.

She accepted responsibility for the mistakes she made due to circumstances she felt necessary at the time. Her daughter was kept safe and was not abused or so she thought. Her daughter was raised in a home provided by her grandmother, a home free of abuse. She made frequent visits to check on her daughter's wellbeing and to take her to school and extracurricular activities. Yet, all the time her daughter contemplated a silent question, "Why don't I live with my mommy?" It plagued her daughter and unfortunately caused a separation of relationship in her daughter's mind as she reached adulthood.

When confronted with the question from her daughter she explained in the best way she could the circumstances surrounding her decision. Her daughter voiced forgiveness, but, the ten year denial for visits to the grandchildren was still enforced.

My client has accepted she will never see her grandchildren and keeps a picture of them on a table next to her bed with pictures of her other grandchildren. It is the last thing she sees at night before she prays and retires to sleep.

Regrets take a toll on the healing process. It is important to keep living. Life never stands still until the heart stops beating. Everyone is capable of forgiving, and if they can't forgive, it is their fault, not yours.

This is an important fact you need to understand. Forgiveness lies in the heart of the person who was hurt by an action. If they cannot find it in their heart to truly forgive – it is their problem. Continue to make up for it as best you can. Live a life of service, kindness, and forgiveness. Sometimes it is all you can do, and in the end, it is up to God to judge our actions not man or woman.

"And when you stand praying, if you hold anything against anyone, forgive him, so that your Father in heaven may forgive you your sins. " Mark 11:25

My client finds comfort in mothering and mentoring young women God places in her path that have poor relationships with their own mothers. She hugs and councils them on how to accept and live with their pain. The affection she receives from those women help to fill the gap, but, her heart weeps for the painful loss of her own daughter's hugs just the same.

MENDING FENCES

There is no time like the present to address broken relationships. It is easier than you may think. What happens when a good friendship or family relationship breaks, and everyone involved refuses to communicate with each other? It pummels the issue forward by days, leading to weeks, leading to months, leading to years, and sometimes a lifetime. It is likened to a train speeding on a track without an engineer. You know the scenario, a silly argument or sudden disagreement ending in hurt and despair leading the ones involved to say harsh things and to disassociate creating a life-long rift.

When this happens, we are in disbelief that our friend or family member has let us down. We believe it is mostly his or her fault, seldom our own. Time goes by and the old friends or family members remain silent. Neither making contact with the other.

Everyone may want reconciliation, but no one will make the first move. They are curious about how the other person is doing, but too angry, embarrassed or ashamed to call. They are afraid to take the risk of re-establishing contact for fear of reopening the old wound.

Sometimes it's pride that keeps them apart, or, just that each party feels that the other was at fault and expects the other person to make the first move. Feelings may be so strong that they never seek reconciliation. Unfortunately, each person in a disagreement or feud only knows their own perspective. The other person's point of view remains a mystery and is confusing to the issue.

For everyone involved in a rift of this magnitude there is a different perspective and understanding of what took place at the specific eventful moment. When we don't know the other person's perspective or unique take on an event, we are at a distinct disadvantage in interpreting what happened

In order to open an exchange of conversation one must also open the old wound. Invite the person to join you. Apologize for your part in the rift regardless of whose fault it was. Offer to listen to their feelings regarding the situation. Communicate without judgment or criticism, only then can healing begin. Listen for the meaning behind the words as you listen to the person talk, and try to understand their perspective on what happened. Do not attack or counter-attack, just listen.

We need to hear the whole story. When they are finished, you can share your thoughts, as long as you do not start another disagreement. Admit your side of being wrong. Apologize and move on. Whatever you do, put the battle to sleep. What really matters is the relationship. No matter how large the rift has become, your relationship or familial tie is what is more important.

Healing your broken relationship begins the moment one person steps up and re-establishes contact, sending a clear message that they care more about the relationship than proving his side of the dispute. Offer a sincere apology and admit you were wrong in some way. Tell the person how important and special they are to you and add you miss them being in your life. A good friend or family member is special! Promise you will not disappoint them in the near future and you'll be there for them.

There is no replacement for a loving friend or family member

Take the initiative to heal the broken relationships in your life. You'll save people a lot of pain - including yourself. One thing to remember, never use your diagnosis of cancer in the conversation as an excuse to heal the relationship. This will send a red flag to the person that you are only mending the broken fence because of your illness.

LETTERS

Saying goodbye is very difficult and in many ways impossible. When I thought my life would be ending sooner than I expected I began preparing my goodbye in the form of letters for my children and grandchildren. Letters they could read after my passing, all the while knowing it would be more painful for them because it is always harder to be the ones left behind than the one to be leaving. I wanted to be sure they were encouraging and happy messages rather than discouraging and sad. It brings to mind a quote I once wrote on a slip of paper and kept as a book marker over the years:

"... Do not be too sad ... You cannot be always torn in two.
You will have to be one and whole, for many years.
You have so much to enjoy and to be, and to do."
                                                            J.R.R. Tolkien

The last thing I wanted to do was crush their spirits by writing anything but precious memories and encouragements for their success in life. I may not have the fortune of being there in person but I assure you I will be cheering for them from the other side.

My heart was filled with a longing so intense I really did not know where and how to begin. I wanted each of them to know how fortunate I was when God blessed me in being their mother.

They were the greatest source of inspiration in my "everyday reason" for living, without even knowing it. I worked hard and focused much my life into the care giving of others and doing the best I could in raising and providing the things my family needed. I was not always right. I made mistakes along the way, but, I loved my children more than life itself. How does one share that in a short letter to cover a lifetime of precious memories?

There are many ways to write letters to say goodbye. The main thing is to write from your heart. If you are writing to someone with whom you have for some reason or another separated from them because of misspoken words in the heat of the moment, or a misplaced blame of some kind make sure you read the chapter on Mending Fences. It can add a wonderful perspective of how to write to them.

Make a list of people for whom you want to write letters. Take time to review your memories of each one. This can be stimulated by looking through family picture albums, special collectables you have harbored as valuable trinkets through the years or anything which stimulates your heart to use when writing your letter to a particular person. Be sure the contents of your letters are all good. Never use a final letter as a way to place blame for anything you are holding a grudge over. Kindness will always win over cruelty, especially when the letter is a remembrance.

I initially wrote individual letters to my three children. Later I thought it best to write a combined letter so they could all know what I had to share with each of them. I upgraded the contents from time to time as they celebrated accomplishments, got married, and had children. I had many letters and many shredded bags as I decided to change the letter one more time. Now that I have published my writings I can toss the original since they will have read the words I have published here for the entire world to see. Then again I may still change the letter as my heart desires – who knows?

A letter to my beloved children, Tammy, Jason, and Joshua,

I remember and cherish the day each of you entered this world. I felt the same excitement, devotion, love, and pride with each of your births. Although the months leading to each of your birth days were very different as life dictates. The days of your births were also different as nature dictates, but, each was very special.

Tammy, you being the first born were my first gift from God and life as a mother. You were a beautiful smiling baby right from the start. Within hours came the frightful news: My exposure to massive radiation in the first trimester of my pregnancy had caused several congenital problems. As the doctor shared all of the things you would have to deal with in your life, including a trip to surgery immediately, burdened my heart, but looking into your bright eyes and awesome smile let me know you were a true fighter and you would overcome all life had dealt you and I knew you would overcome everything with God's help.

Jason, you came along ten years later. Oh how I wanted twin girls on Valentine's Day – but God had different plans. I did not know whether you were a boy or a girl but I was assured there was only one baby. The week before you were born you decided to take a siesta. You stopped moving. I thought I was carrying a dead child within me and I was scared to death if you were alive you would be born with congenital problems and each day brought forth new imaginations of horrible defects in the form of nightmares as I slept. I had been in contact with the doctor every day for seven days and by this time I had worried him there may be a problem.

So I went to the doctor's office and was rushed into the examining room. Well let me tell you all heck broke loose. You were done napping! As I entered the exam room my water broke and I screamed! What a mess! Slipping out of my clothes and waddling across the hall with a paper sheet wrapped around me was all I could do to save face as curious onlookers watched the calamity unfold.

Needless to say, I was in labor and you were almost delivered in the car before I got to the hospital which was less than two miles from the doctor's office. You had been playing possum very well. You just had to make sure you came quick and with little warning. I remember in the delivery room bombarding the staff with questions about your condition. I was so fearful you would have congenital problems as your sister had, but, the only thing they found as they examined you after birth was – you were tongue tied and they clipped it a few days after you were born and that was that. Not to mention you were born the day before Valentine's Day and most definitely you were not twin girls! This is something I will never regret. You were my first born son and I loved you just the same.

Joshua, you came 20 months after your brother. Do you remember my saying if you had been born first you would probably have been the last? Not because I did not love you but I swear you were born with roller skates on your feet and never needed sleep. For the first year you never slept more than two hours a day. To this day I do not know how I kept my sanity.

I remember when you were two years old I put a lock on the top of the door to the outside because you would wait till I was asleep and you would sneak outside to play. Once I could not find you in the morning and the door was still locked as well as all of the window sills. I found you on the top of a kitchen cupboard against the ceiling sound asleep. You had taken a chair, climbed onto the counter, stacked a tray on the toaster and up you went to the top of the cupboard near the refrigerator where the bird cage sat. I can only assume you were talking to the birds, climbed to the top to be closer and fell asleep.

God was faithful and I was blessed. Tammy, you were more than I could have imagined a daughter to be. As a young child you were headstrong, determined, and gifted. You were determined to overcome all obstacles to refute the doctors forecast for your future. You not only overcame their dismal forecasts you excelled in every way as you matured and are so gifted in many ways.

Jason, you have always been my intuitive child – it must be because you are what they classify as the middle child! You tended to be more quiet and listened to everything including the breeze, Because of that special way of communication you have a deep understanding and connection with the souls of others much like me. You are so giving of yourself and give even when you have little to share. God will bless you for this my son – it is a service not all are capable of.

Joshua, you were always the suborned one. The stubborn part I grew to understand as your "special touch" with the world, because you always had a way of doing things your way – even if it was wrong – it worked out for you. Remember the time you cut the wires from Jason's new stereo speakers so you could have longer wires for your own? I can laugh about it today but at the time I was so angry. You had not considered your brother's feelings at all, but, today I see the ingenuity of your active mind in creating something new.

To all of you I want to say how much I cherished all of the trips in the car as you were growing up whether it was for swimming events, twirling lessons, twirling competitions, dance classes, parades, baseball games, track meets, football games, band practice, band nights, or award banquets and everything involved in your growing up I may have missed mentioning. Those times spent in the car with you bring such wonderful memories to my heart. The hundreds of trophies, medals, awards, citations, pictures, high school diplomas, and college degrees which graced our home were my pride in your accomplishments.

The spouses you have chosen are a complement to your personality and of your choosing. I am proud of what you have accomplished as parents: All of the grandchildren – the yours, mine, ours, and adopted are all equal in my heart and it makes me so proud of the legacy you are leaving in this family.

Tammy and Scott, you could not have done better raising your children in faith which is your chosen career. Josiah, Charis, and Faith are beautiful, intelligent, children and such a testament with their faithfulness to God.

Jason, I am so proud of how you have stepped up and are giving Bridgette's children Brian, Coty, and Anissa, a father. You have raised and guided them in life and faith and I honor and respect your maintaining them safely in your loving arms.

Joshua, to raise two sons as a single parent is quite an accomplishment and I have seen you mature in patience and understanding as the years have passed and I take pride as you have grown in responsibility and given Joshua, Jr and Conner a stable home. I am also proud of the relationship you have with Deanna and the combined family you have created taking Corey, Kyle, and Casey as your own.

As I sit on the back deck in the sunlight feeling its warmth on my skin as I write this letter I let my mind wander over the years passed and smile remembering so many wonderful times I have spent being your mother. I want you to know how you have touched my life in a way nothing else in this world could. I love you so very much. Please do not mourn my passing. It is important you remember I have always said, "I have my bags packed and I am *ready when God calls me home." I have visited once and I will be there when you are called to join me. Love my grandchildren as I have loved you. Honor them and nourish them in the word of God.*

Now, go out and celebrate my passing. Know I am in the arms of God. Enjoy the lessons I have left for you; laugh, love, and enjoy what our life has meant to each other.

All of my love, forever, and into eternity,
Mom

FAITH AND MY DECISION TO FOREGO TREATMENT

On a day to day basis it is rare we contemplate the length of our lives or the circumstances surrounding our time of death. From the day we are born we have a time on this earth living a life we have chosen to live. However, receiving a terminal diagnosis has a way of putting many things into a different perspective and in the forefront of our conscious thoughts. Some will reflect on the life they have lived while others will center their thoughts on loved ones and the time they have left to spend with them. Life itself will be viewed in a different light by each and every one of us. Many may turn to the faith they currently practice or reconnect with early life religious teachings. The challenges associated with cancer or any debilitating disease leads a person to search, connect, and find solace in an inner strength. Peace and encouragement from any entity that gives a person encouragement in their time of need will add a positive component to the healing process.

Churches, synagogues, temples, spiritual leaders, faith, and support groups in general can be a great resource for patients dealing with a terminal illness. Patients who turn to their faith and spiritual beliefs are able to restore their strength and sometimes gain a deeper love and understanding about their life's journey.

Supportive services within religious communities provide organized support for the patient and their family. Simple emotional comfort can change the lives of everyone involved by instilling a peace and understanding as they embrace the battle of a critical illness encroaching on their lives.

When I have a need for healing I pray for the Creator to heal my body as He sees fit. As much as I want to be specific in my prayers I don't know what His plans are for me or for my life. Of course I want to live a long healthy life. I want to be able to continue to be a caregiver, offering help to the sick, and encourage them in their time of need. I want to be able to share the importance of forgiveness, of being non-judgmental, and of harboring no prejudice, the life teachings that have been so important to me in my lifetime.

I am a believer. I have learned the more you are in good favor of others, the more you are beloved by God. When I say this I am not referring to popularity or number of friends you have, but, being in good favor of others is being admired for the good life example you set for others. Be diligent in living an exemplary life. Even in illness carry God in your heart and on your face.

It is important to learn to be silent and speak what is true and worth hearing. My habit of sharing my faith in subtle ways is a way to plant seeds in the listener's heart and mind. Truths and soft words have a magic effect on the receiver. I may never see those seeds come to fruition and bear fruit but I plant the seeds all the same.

This is not to say I have not been angry with God. I have been! There was an occasion when I could not bear one more thing. My life was unraveling. Both of my parents were dying of cancer. I was taking care of my mother who was bedfast at home while my father was in an extended care facility in a coma. I was working full time in an Intensive Care Unit giving all I could manage to give to help the critically ill patients assigned to my care and trying to hold together an extremely broken marriage.

On this particular day, I was knee deep in my own pain and devastation, but, it was part of my job to approach families of brain dead patients for permission to harvest organs for transplant. It was one part of my job I dreaded. Even though it was a responsibility I had to fulfill, the need to comfort those in my care was never an issue for me no matter what my personal situation was at that moment. Their needs always came first many times at the cost of my family needs.

I had spoken the words to request organs for harvesting many times in my career, but, this time it hit home as I approached a single mother, losing her only child, by telling her his death would not be in vain should she decide to donate his organs to save or improve the lives of others. She sat for a long time, tears flowing freely as I held her in my arms. She then looked up and said, "What would you do?"

As tears flowed from my eyes I choked out the words, "I have always taught my children to do the best they could for others as long as they are in this world. As hard as it would be to know it meant I would lose my child in this life, I would allow them to harvest their organs, knowing there was no greater gift for them to give than life."

She signed the transplant harvest papers and the team was called. I stayed with her through the procedure and she was allowed to say goodbye to her only child. I held her, cried with her, and comforted her in her pain until she was able to leave the hospital that day.

As I drove home I continued to cry as my heart broke for the pain she must be feeling. As I turned into my driveway my own reality struck like a bolt of lightning. To add to my burden, I remembered running into my doctor earlier that morning as I hand carried blood to the lab. He took me aside and gave me the results of my recent mammogram. The mammogram verified I had a walnut size tumor in my breast. I had discovered the lump at five o'clock on my left breast two weeks earlier and the doctor had discovered five palpable lymph nodes under my left arm a few days after.

I entered the door of my home holding back the sobs crushing to heave from my chest. I knew the result before he uttered the words, but, hearing it from his lips confirmed it was a death sentence for me. Anger boiled within my heart. I slammed the door and screamed and screamed again. I threw my work bag down the basement stairs in a rage and raised my hands toward the ceiling. I yelled at God, "You are my Father and you are supposed to take care of me. Why are you not taking care of me? I am tired and can't take any more. I am done. If this is what having a Father in heaven is like I am not sure I want a Father anymore!"

My body slumped to the floor and I cried until I was drained of tears. I asked over and over, "Why Lord? Why?" Feeling totally spent with no more energy to question God, I rose and felt my body pinned softly to the door.

A life review flashed through my mind as though someone had created a movie of my life. I saw my childhood memories, my graduation, the birth of my children, my career and suddenly I felt the warmth of God's love wrap around me as my mind cleared. I realized my parents needed me to take care of them and I had to remain strong. My personal health had to be put aside. My needs were unimportant. I knew I would do what I had to do and I would live with the consequences of my decisions.

I was thankful my daughter was safe at college and my sons were playing in the back yard very much alive and not waiting to have a machine turned off ending their time on earth any time soon. I moved slowly up the stairs, through the kitchen, and out the back door. I grabbed a hoe from the barn and headed to the garden. Beating up weeds taking over my garden was one way I worked through problems bearing down on my heart, but, usually I did not do it in my work uniform. I heard my older son say to his younger brother, "Something happened at work. Don't bother mom right now." He had a gift of insight and intuition from a very young age and always seemed to know when something was not right with me.

I noticed him sitting under a tree nearby watching me as I worked between the plants pulling the wild weeds and drawing fresh earth up around the stems of each plant. I had chopped through a few rows in the garden and had worked through the decision making the ache in my chest hurt a little less. That was it. My decision was made! I would not have surgery to remove the tumor in my breast and I would not have chemotherapy or radiation. I had seen what the treatments had done to my mother. The treatments had stolen quality time from her as the treatments killed the good cells with the bad.

When I put the hoe into the barn the boys came together and hugged me. They wanted to know why I went to the garden. We sat under a tree near the garden as I shared the heart breaking story of the young man I had cared for that day but I held back telling them their own mother had a cancerous lump in her breast. They had enough to digest with the every day events surrounding the changes in their Grandmother's journey.

Maintaining our faith walk is a constant challenge in good times and even harder when we are facing troubled times in our lives. We read scriptures and teachings of the apostles and yet how are we to understand and apply the message and its power to our lives as we live in this century. This was the first time I made the connection: "Why not me?" instead of "Why me?"

As a believer, I trusted God even if I got upset with His decisions regarding our lives I trusted Him. A few weeks after this event my mother began having difficulty breathing. The radiation treatments had burnt her neck and chest severely. A huge swelling appeared on the front of her neck, pressing against and narrowing her wind pipe. As she struggled to breathe, I called her oncologist who was unavailable. I then called her primary care physician. He said to bring her into his office for an exam.

As I helped my mother dress I bargained with God. I had made the declaration to God on that fateful day I beat the weeds to death in my garden to decline western medical cancer treatments, but this did not stop me from trying to make a deal with God in regards to my Mother's wellbeing. I looked at the huge swelling preventing my mother's intake of breath, all the time thinking she would have to have a tracheotomy placed if it grew any bigger. As I buttoned her blouse I asked God to give the ugly swollen mass to me. I told Him I was younger, stronger, and more equipped to handle the pain. I begged Him to keep me well enough to see my mother through her illness and pledged I would accept whatever He had planned for me if only He would rid her of the huge mass blocking her airway and make her comfortable.

We went to the physician's office and he took an x-ray of her neck. It showed a soft tissue mass which was causing a shift in her airway. It was not caused from the burn. It was a metastatic growth of the disease. He gave her a heavy dose of prednisone and asked to see her again the following morning. The plan was to give her time to digest the three options available for treatment. The first option was to have the mass surgically removed. The second option was to have a tracheotomy placed to allow her to breathe around the mass, and the third option was to do nothing and allow the cancer to run its course.

My mother understood everything the doctor said and was silently contemplating on the drive home. I was engrossed in my discussion with God. I continued to ask Him to give the mass to me. That night I slept in a rocking chair in my mother's room. I wanted to be sure I was nearby if she struggled to breath. I awakened early the next morning and noticed my mother's breathing was normal. As I leaned closer to listen I felt a sharp pain run across the right side of my sternum into my neck. I pulled my shirt open and saw a red swelling about the size of an egg. I could not believe it. God had answered my prayer. I began to cry. I was of so little faith at times, but, God had heard my prayer and had answered my plea.

I did not say anything to my Mother as we prepared to go to the doctor that morning. I waited for the doctor's response when he examined her neck. He said he had never seen anything like it. He had another x-ray taken and the soft tissue mass was not evident in the film. As he examined the images side by side he shook his head.

I said, "You need to look at my neck."

He asked with a slightly sarcastic tone of chiding, "Why do you need to be checked?"

I explained. "I asked God to give me the mass." He chuckled freely as he checked my neck and when he felt the warm raised lump the smile on his face changed to concern. He insisted it was not possible to bargain with God and I must have developed an abscess or an inflamed lymph node from my own breast tumor.

Forgetting my mother was present, I reminded him, "My tumor is on the left breast and the inflamed swelling is on the right breast, chest, and neck. I asked him if he was in the mindset that I now had tumors on both breasts."

He angrily instructed me, "God does not give the afflictions of one person to another no matter how hard we pray. Have the secretary schedule a mammogram on the other breast as soon as possible." I did not bother.

The drive home was a silent one. My Mother did not know I

had developed a tumor in my breast. She was angry I had not shared the information with her and she had to hear it from the doctor. I had intentionally kept it from her. I felt it would only add stress to an already stressful situation. I explained to her as she remained silent I had been reading articles about cancer being treated with dietary changes and decided to forgo the current treatment options and would seek someone to help me heal the tumor with diet. I assured her this thing on my neck and chest would be gone in a few days and miraculously it was.

MY NEAR DEATH EXPERIENCE

I was 37 years old. I had been hemorrhaging off and on for months and physicians made decisions based on symptoms and lab results. There were no amazing imaging machines to show them what was going on within a body like a CAT scan or an MRI. I initially had a minor procedure called a D&C where they cleaned the lining of the uterus. Pathology results returned positive with three pre-cancer cells in varying degrees of maturity. The pathologist explained if I did not have a hysterectomy I would have "full blown" cancer within six months. With this news I agreed and had the hysterectomy in early 1986. The procedure went well and I was recovering at home when we had an earthquake in Northeast Ohio, on January 31st measuring 5.0 on the Richter scale. It literally threw dishes out of the China cabinet and dropped pictures hanging on the wall to the floor. Within an hour I was having severe pain in my right side. The pain was so intense I had to lie down. Three hours following the earthquake I was taken to the emergency room and readmitted to the hospital with unexplainable abdominal pain. After several days of x-rays and testing, I turned bright neon yellow-green. I was jaundiced. My Obstritician consulted a General Surgeon. Further testing found a large stone in the biliary tree. The stone was too large to pass into the common bile duct causing a back up of bile which had a toxic life threatening effect on my body.

I spent six weeks in the hospital and they made five surgical attempts to remove the stone, but, each time they tried to get near the stone wedged in the biliary tree I would hemorrhage and they would have to stop.

I was sent home with several drains planted into my abdomen and a plethora of medications to control infection and pain. I was unable to eat without severe nausea and vomiting. I had lost a quarter of my body weight and had salt crystal deposits on my skin which I was shedding like a snake. My abdomen looked like I was nine months pregnant and all of my medications were liquid. I was awaiting admission to a major medical center for assessment of a possible liver transplant. It was now nearing the end of March.

The volume of prescribed medication for my pain was low. There was not enough for another dose. My uncle went to the pharmacy and had it refilled. The pharmacist did not tell my uncle the medication strength was double the prescribed dose and I should only take half of the amount previously ordered. The bottle was the same color, shape, and size as previously dispensed. The first rule of nursing is to verify a medication by its label and its dose. I never failed to do this on the job but here I was at home in severe pain and had just poured a lethal dose of pain killer that would stop my ability to breath.

Within minutes I felt a strange feeling of impending doom. Somehow I knew I was in trouble. I managed to drag myself to the bathroom. I thought I was going to throw up, but, I realized I could not breathe. I tried to scream but no sound passed my lips.

In a moments time I was no longer in my body. I was formless and hovering at the ceiling watching my body fall to the floor. I watched blood stream from my forehead where it had struck the counter of the sink. The next thing I remember was screaming, "Lord, I'm not done yet, I have kids to raise."

As I begged not to die I realized I no longer had form. I felt whole. I felt alive more alive than I had for months. In an instant I was encompassed by a warm, bright, golden light, and I could feel an overwhelming presence of a community of others like myself. I was greeted with a sharing of all knowing wisdom, kindness, compassion and intelligence. It was like a fountain being poured into my mind. My senses heightened even though I had no form. I was greeted without speech yet I was communicating fully. I felt such love and acceptance within the community. I smelled fragrances greater than any flower I had ever smelled on earth. I experienced colors I had never seen before. My questions were answered before I even asked them. Most of all I felt the presence of God as the golden cloak of light encompassed me from behind as though someone wrapped a warm blanket around me. I felt a presence of the Spirit of God. I felt a wisp of air grace my cheek as His lips spoke into my right ear, "Have no fear my child. It's not your time." In the next moment I was back in my pain wracked body.

What is important is I did not share this out of body experience with anyone for many years. I searched and searched in books for answers. I read books about other religions. I read all I could get my hands on about "Near Death Experiences." As much as I did not want to die and leave my children, I felt somehow maybe I was not good enough to stay in the presence of God. I felt unworthy.

Many years later when I opened my heart to share my experience with one of my College Professors she said to me, "Stop it! Stop it now! Stop questioning God's reasoning and just accept the fact you are precious to Him and this is why your heart beats today." From that moment in time I have had my bags packed just in case today could be the day He calls for me. I am ready.

Know and accept there is an afterlife. I have been there. It is a place with God, of God, and about God. No matter how you call Him; Lord of Lords; King of Kings; Christ; Jesus; Waheguru; Elohim; Jehova; Yahweh; Dio; Mio Dio; The Great I AM; or by any other religious name of faith as long as you believe there is a God and you accept Him as your Father. There is a place where other souls join together, a place of peace, tranquility, knowledge, and harmony, a place called Heaven. Don't let the opportunity escape you. Open your heart today and accept God as your Savior. You don't want to miss out on it - there is a Heaven!

LAYING ON OF HANDS

The Laying on of hands has been practiced since Biblical times. Although it is not practiced in all religions it is still practiced by many of faith today. All believers have the privilege to lay hands on the sick and I do not believe it is limited to the gifted.

Having faith in our Creator and the belief He can heal the sick is all it takes. Anyone can lay hands on themselves. God uses us as a vessel for His Spirit and also as a tool in which to deliver the healing power of His Spirit through an act of faith. Most healers place their hands on a person's head but I choose to allow the Spirit of God to lead me to where my hands must lay. Many times I ask the person if it is comfortable for them if I touch them where I plan to seek Gods healing before I lay hands on them.

The healing power of God through the laying on of hands transfers the power of God through His spirit to enter the body which needs healing. I believe in seeking God's presence in the moment before I actively lay hands on someone through prayer. I seek His blessings, His plan for the soul, and His will be done within the person I am seeking healing for.

I pray softly near the receiver's ear so they can hear my praise of our Father God and my request for specific healing for them. I lay my hands upon the area where the sickness lies placing it in between my hands. If the sickness lies in an area of personal nature I place my hands over the person's heart front and back and ask God to remove all obstacles blocking the way of healing and the removal of sickness from the body.

I know my body reacts to my prayers before I lay my hands on a person. I feel the Spirit of God take over. I feel the energy of God's presence and I even sweat at times because the energy is so over powering. Heat emanates from my body.

A young woman in New York City asked me if I was a healer after hearing me speak to a group of conference attendees about my Coaching practice. Her question caught me off guard and I quickly answered, "No." I saw disappointment flush over her face as she heard my answer. I quickly reached for her hand and said, "Wait... wait... I am only a vessel and God is the healer." I whispered, "What is your need?" I saw tears welling in her eyes as she told me about the discovery of a lump in her left breast. I said meet me following the conference and I will lay hands on you in the name of God's spirit.

The conference was closed with quiet meditation and while the speaker was bringing the audience to a sacred place I was asking God to fill me with His spirit to lay hands on the young woman filled with fear sitting across the table from me. I reached to grasp the hand of those believers sitting beside me and as we closed our fingers together I lifted our clasped hands onto the tabletop in plain view. Those two women followed my lead taking the next persons hand and the others followed suit as it created a circle of women connected.

The conference was not a spiritual conference but somehow we at that table knew it was a spiritual alliance for us because all but one seated at our table were believers. There was one non-believer sitting with us but she amazingly took part in our lunchtime prayer as we prayed the blessing of our food and by adding her hands to the group closing the circle. I felt God's presence grow as I prayed for His Spirit to fill me. I felt the women on both sides of me loosen their grip as my hands heated, but they continued to hold close. Immediately following the close of meditation the conference leader wished us well and the circle of women let go of each of the others hands.

I made eye contact and nodded at the young woman and she ran to my side of the table. As I moved chairs to make space for the two of us she hugged me tightly before I even spoke. After our hug I took her hands and ask if I could place one hand over her left breast above her heart and one on her back. She agreed and I brought her close to me so I could pray softly into her ear. She hugged me tightly as the Holy Spirit of God took over and I began to pray for her healing according to God's will. The Spirit filled me as I praised God and asked His blessing on the young woman. I prayed for some time holding her tightly as the Spirit moved. When I felt the Spirit of God empty from my body to hers I let her know, praying for healing and laying on of hands is a spiritual request and does not guarantee healing for her, but, it is whatever God's will is for her life that is important. She voiced understanding and acceptance.

The entire table of believers and the non-believer made a circle of prayer. One of the women in our group spoke to God asking His blessings for the group of women who had been led to sit at the same table. I intentionally stood next to the non-believer and laid my hand on the left side of her back behind where her heartbeat could be felt beneath my fingertips as I prayed for a special healing and opening of her mind. I also asked God to send someone into her active life who could influence her about God's presence. She was placed in our group for a reason. She was not a believer, not an alumnus from our school, nor was she a Holistic Health Coach.

I fully believe: Nothing happens by coincidence – It is God's way of remaining anonymous. We were placed together for the future and we have yet to see it unfold in God's time.

If one has the faith God can heal, they can pray asking God to allow the Holy Spirit to enter the body and remove the illness. Faith is all it takes, a faith in God's ability to answer prayer. God's power is amazing. He can heal the sick and make the blind see. Trust Him and ask for healing according to His will.

COMPLIMENTARY AND ALTERNATIVE CHOICES

Herbal supplements are a matter of personal choice but it is imperative you seek guidance from a reliable source before making a decision to stop conventional treatment. Don't follow the path of a magazine article recently published until you have thoroughly researched the data and spoken with an expert in the field of treatment offered. Discontinuation of prescribed antineoplastic agents can be a very tricky process.

Everyone needs to understand alternative treatments are less studied. This does not mean they can't be affective – it means they are unproven except through those who have made the leap and spoken about it like myself and those involved in Dr. Kelly Turner's study about Radical Remissions.

Unless you have an Ayurvedic practitioner or a Naturopathic physician who is trained in the use of supplements, I would not opt to discontinue prescribed medications. However, there are safe supplements for specific uses and can be used in place of prescribed medications, if they are effective for you. For example: Supplements for cleanses and detoxification are safe to use in conjunction with prescribed medications, but, you should consult your physician prior to discontinuing any medication he has prescribed.

Medications for specific medical issues such as high blood pressure, heart conditions, and diabetes should never be replaced with supplements unless prescribed by a licensed practitioner. This could cause irreparable damage to the health of your system.

Ayurveda emphasizes prevention of disease, individualization of treatment, and maintenance of balance between body, mind, and spirit. The approach can be considered appropriate in most clinical circumstance and is considered as such in India. Ayurvedic doctors will spend time diagnosing a patient's overall health and resilience, including an assessment of which organ systems are functioning appropriately versus which ones are weak. Mental status as well as the level of life-energy is assessed in detail. Understanding a person's constitution is unchanging, but their interaction with the environment around them can cause dynamic imbalances.

The role Vitamin D plays in cell development and the fact that so many people are deficient in Vitamin D has brought it to the forefront as an additional supplement for cancer patients recently and it has stirred interest for much needed research into its plausible effect on cancer and healing.

Garlic and onions should be consumed daily in any form; raw, powdered, or cooked. Substances found in garlic and onions have been shown to suppress growth and fight certain cancerous cells in the lab, including forms of breast and lung cancer.

Turmeric, an Indian spice readily used in cooking of many vegetable dishes contains curcumin which is considered to be an active antioxidant which demonstrates anti-cancer effects. According to the American Cancer Society Turmeric is particularly effective in slowing growth of tumors of the esophagus, mouth, intestines, stomach, breast, and skin. Turmeric is an anti-inflammatory herbal remedy and is said to produce fewer side effects than common pain relievers. Some practitioners prescribe turmeric to relieve inflammation caused by arthritis, muscle sprains, swelling, and pain caused by injuries or surgical incisions.

It is also promoted as a treatment for rheumatism and as an antiseptic for cleaning wounds.
http://www.cancer.org/treatment/treatmentsandsideeffects/complementaryandalternativemedicine/herbsvitaminsandminerals/turmeric

Matcha and Oolong teas contain powerful substances called polyphenols that are believed to have powerful anti-cancer abilities. One glass of Matcha tea has ten times the healing power of Oolong tea. Cancerous tumors rely on fast-growing networks of blood vessels to sustain their rapid growth rate know as angiogenesis. Green tea compounds may possess the ability to help slow or prevent this rapid growth which inhibits the development of new blood vessels in tumors.

Matcha tea is an antioxident powerhouse. It detoxifies effectively and naturally, calms and relaxes , enhances mood and aids in concentration, provides vitamin C, selenium, chromium, zinc and magnesium, fights against viruses and bacteria, is rich in fiber, lowers cholesterol and blood sugar, and does not raise insulin levels. It contains EGCg and other catechins which counteract the effects of free radicals from GMOs, radiation, and chemicals, which can lead to cell and DNA damage. Visit lordimnotdoneyet.com for more information and where to buy the best quality Matcha tea.

Antioxidants are substances found in abundance in fruits and vegetables. Phytochemicals fight certain oxygen molecules in your body known as free radicals, which can damage DNA and contribute to the development and proliferation of cancerous cells. Common antioxidants include selenium, vitamins A, C, E, and certain compounds found in green tea.

Ginger is one of the best anti nausea treatments available for nausea and vomiting which are the most common side effects of chemotherapy and can be brewed in a tea to be used for nausea and vomiting. These side effects can be serious. Nausea and vomiting can lead to weight loss, nutritional deficiencies, and fatigue, which can make it harder for your body to fight cancer. There are a number of anti-nausea medications available. But some patients with cancer also find that using ginger; either alone or in conjunction with anti-nausea medicine, significantly reduces nausea and vomiting.

Mangosteen is a tropical fruit native to Southeast Asia that is touted for its antioxidants, especially xanthones. There are documented studies which show apoptosis and antioxidative actions of mangosteen as published in 2003 by Elsavier Ireland Ltd via mangosteenmd.org. On the other hand, according to the American Cancer Society, there is no reliable evidence that mangosteen juice, puree, or bark is effective as a treatment for cancer in humans. Its fruit has been shown to be rich in anti-oxidants. Early small laboratory and animal studies suggest that further research should be done to determine whether it can help to prevent cancer in humans.

http://www.cancer.org/treatment/treatmentsandsideeffects/complementaryandalternativemedicine/pharmacologicalandbiological treatment/mangosteen-juice

Detox Bath

A bath is one of the best healthy fit therapies we can experience to facilitate our body's natural detoxification system of the skin. There is no doubt our bodies are subjected to many toxins daily. Toxins are in the air we breathe, the food we eat, in the water we drink, and in the homes we live in. Toxins cause irritation, harm, and destruction in bodily function if left unchecked. Detoxification is the body's way of removing and metabolizing toxic compounds. Detoxification is done naturally and reflexively without our awareness through our liver, kidneys, digestive system, and skin.

Metabolic waste from toxins build up in our body causing malfunction and illness. The liver removes this waste and toxins from the body by converting them to water-soluble compounds. Once water-soluble they can be eliminated from the body through urine. Some waste products are not water-soluble and are transformed by the liver and excreted in the bile. The bile is then transported to the intestines where it exits the body through our digestive system. Toxins not eliminated or completely removed by either of these processes may be eliminated through our skin via sweat.

In addition to removing toxins a detox bath can:
- Ease stress
- Improve sleep
- Improve concentration
- Help muscles and nerves function properly
- Reduce inflammation
- Relieve pain
- improve exchange of oxygen in the cells
- Improve absorption of nutrients
- Open pores and allow escape of toxins via sweat
- Aids in exfoliation of dead skin cells

Colonic Detoxification – Rectal

There are many theories pro and con regarding detoxification and use of colonics. First let me give you a simple explanation of our digestive process. Our salivary glands secrete digestive juices as we chew our food. Once swallowed, the stomach releases specific acids, churns the food to aid digestion, and sends it into the intestinal system.

Intestines are responsible for the digestion and elimination of food we eat. The digestive process is to extract the nutritional value from the food we consume and eliminate the left over useless trash through the evacuation of stool. Our bowels act as a storage reservoir for the processed waste until it is evacuated from the body.

Each person has different bowel function related to the diet they consume, the amount of water they drink, and the level of their daily exercise. People with sluggish bowels or those who experience frequent constipation can hold several pounds of fecal waste which tends to break down the interior bowel causing further chronic problems.

Blockages can occur from the sluggish or constipated bowel many times requiring painful extraction procedures to bowel obstructions requiring surgical procedures. Other problems related to but not limited to unhealthy bowels are hemorrhoids, IBS - irritable bowel syndrome, colitis, Crohn's disease, obesity, and many others.

The bowel serves as the body's first line of defense through its bacteria which identifies and eliminates viruses and unhealthy materials we have ingested with our food. Colonic detoxification procedures provide an effective fecal cleansing of the colon as well as providing effective herbal combinations which will sooth and heal the mucous membrane lining of the intestinal tract. The combined action of this type of colonic detoxification also cleanses the liver through stimulation of bile production and does not contain any habit forming compounds.

Colonic detoxification will reduce gas, sooth and heal the intestine and allow for improved function of liver, gall bladder, and intestine and is usually done through oral ingestion or administration of an enema via the rectum.

Colonics using specific herbal combination of coffee, or tea, are generally administered rectally and are used for cleansing of liver and colon for cancer patients. It is generally used to remove toxins from the body introduced through chemotherapy and to reduce pain.

I do a coffee colonic twice weekly because I do not have a gall bladder and my bile drips in small amounts continually into my bowel as it is produced rather than when I need food digested. I also use Psyllium husks to aid motility in my bowel. I place a teaspoon in a glass of juice in the morning and it aids in the movement of waste through the bowel and keeps liquid stool in a gelatin form and softens constipated stool for easier evacuation.

Colonic Detoxification – Oral

Oral Colonic Detoxification programs are usually a balanced herbal treatment taken over a designated number of days. Some require fasting with exception of water while others allow specified dietary intake. These procedures should be discussed with your physician to assure they are safe for you to use.

Juice Fast

Dr Andrew Weil, Founder & Director of the Arizona Center for Integrative Medicine at the University of Arizona College of Medicine, suggests a daylong or weekend "juice fast" plus some powdered psyllium seed husks to give your intestines bulk. A juice fast can be healthful and is simple to do:

Juice: Drink at least four 8 - to 12-ounce glasses of juice daily, plus at least four 8-ounce glasses of water and, if you like, some unsweetened herbal tea. If possible, prepare the juice yourself from organically grown fruits and vegetables. One combination I like is apple, carrot and lemon juice, diluted with plain or sparkling water. If you can't make your own juices, buy natural ones without added sugar and dilute them to taste with water.

Psyllium seed: Stir one tablespoon of psyllium powder (available at health food stores) into a big glass of water, drink it, and then drink another glass of plain water. Do this once a day, preferably in the morning.

He further suggests: While you fast, take 100 mg of vitamin C twice a day, but skip your other supplements. (http://www.drweilblog.com/home/2011/3/22/the-best-cleanse.html)

COPING WITH THE SIDE EFFECTS OF TREATMENT

Nausea is the most common side effect of cancer treatments and many times creates additional problems as the body fails to replenish its fuel supply provided by dietary intake.

Suggestions for Coping with nausea

- Sit upright when eating and remain upright for at least one hour following meals
- Eat small meals often and eat slowly
- Eat foods at room temperature or chilled foods rather than hot foods.
- Snack on crackers, toast, or unseasoned salad croutons.
- Avoid foods that are fried, spicy, or, those having a strong odor.
- Sip on clear liquids such as Matcha, ginger, or cardamom teas, broth, or frozen fruit cubes to prevent dehydration.
- If you are on chemo therapy rinse your mouth with baking soda and salt before and after meals, 1 quart water, ¾ teaspoon salt and 1 teaspoon baking soda.
- If there is a bad taste in your mouth chew a ¼ teaspoon of fennel seeds mixed with mint flavored sprinkles after rinsing.

- Anti-nausea medications can be added at the discretion of your physician.

Natural Recipes for Soothing GI Upset

Recipe - Puréed Fennel Soup

Sauté 1 1/2 pounds trimmed and chopped fennel and 1 peeled and chopped onion in 2 tablespoons Ghee to soften, about 5 minutes. Add 5 cups stock or water and bring to a boil. Cover the pot, lower the heat and simmer until fennel is tender, about 15-20 minutes. Cool, place in Vita Mixer (or blender) and puree, strain and refrigerate. Serve chilled. This is also good to sip on when nauseated.

Recipe - Chilled Melon Soup

In a bowl, whisk together 2 cups vanilla yogurt, 1/4 cup milk, ½ tsp cardamom. In another bowl, combine the grated flesh of a ripe medium cantaloupe melon, 2 tablespoons Agave nectar or date syrup; refrigerate bowls for 2 hours, stirring once. To serve, spoon yogurt onto melon and stir. Serve chilled.

Recipe - Puréed Carrot Soup

Sauté 1 1/2 pounds diced carrots and 1 chopped onion in 2 tablespoons Ghee to soften, about 5 minutes. Add 5 cups vegetable or chicken stock, 1 tsp salt, 1 tsp turmeric, and bring to a boil. Cover, lower the heat, and simmer until carrots are tender, about 15 minutes. Cool. Purée in Vita mixer or blender and refrigerate. Garnish with fresh chopped Cilantro. Serve chilled.

Recipe - Watermelon Gazpacho

Combine 1/2 pound finely chopped tomatoes (skin removed)

with 1 1/2 pounds seeded and finely cubed watermelon, 1 peeled and finely diced cucumber (seeds removed,) 3 Tablespoons olive oil, 1/2 tsp turmeric, ½ tsp cardamom, 2 Tablespoons Agave Nectar or date syrup in a food processor or blender; process until chunky-smooth. Serve chilled over finely cubed watermelon.

How to Brew Oolong Tea

Use a high-quality, good-tasting water. This is crucial to produce good tea.

- Use the right amount of loose tea leaves. When brewing loose leaf oolong tea, you should use about one heaping teaspoon of leaves per eight ounces of water. This produces good tasting brewed tea, which is not too strong or weak. Use more or less oolong leaves, depending on your preferences.
- Use boiling water. Unlike some other more fragile teas, such as green tea and white tea, oolong leaves are sturdy enough to withstand boiling water. For a true, full-flavored oolong tea, use boiling water when brewing.
- Allow the tea to brew for the correct length of time. As a general rule of thumb, you should allow loose leaf oolong tea leaves steep for about three to five-minutes, and no longer. Allowing the tea to steep longer than this will produce a cup that is too bitter to drink. Try brewing for three minutes, and if you desire a stronger tasting tea, allow the oolong leaves to steep longer next time.

Some tea experts advise against adding milk or sweeteners to oolong tea, as the flavors do not compliment the flavor of the tea. You should try drinking your brewed oolong plain at least once before you decide to add other ingredients to your cup of tea. Steeping tea for Steeping tea for at least five minutes releases the most antioxidants. The grade of the tea and the time of its harvest will also influence the appropriate steeping temperature. Green teas picked earlier in the spring will benefit from lower temperature brewing due to their overall higher levels of amino acids.

Recipe - Indian Cardamom tea

Lightly crush 7 green cardamom pods so the seeds are exposed. Place the pods, ½" cube of fresh ginger, 4 whole cloves and 1 cinnamon stick in a small pot and cover with 1 cup of water and bring to a slow boil for around 10 minutes. Add 3 cups of milk (coconut, almond, rice milk can be substituted for whole milk) and 3 heaping teaspoons black tea. I use Lipton Yellow label or Darjeeling tea. Keep on a very low heat so that the milk scalds but does not boil. Steep the tea for about 10 minutes. Add Agave Nectar or Date Syrup to taste or sweetener of your choice. Pour through a strainer into cups and enjoy!

How to Brew Matcha tea

Machta tea is the only tea where the entire leaf is consumed. It delivers the highest grade of nutritional benefits and is high in antioxidant activity which offers protection against many kinds of cancer. It helps prevent cardiovascular disease and slows the aging process. It also helps reduce harmful cholesterol in the blood, stabilizes blood sugar levels, and enhances resistance of the body to many toxins. It is the simplest tea to make. It can be sipped hot or cold and can be enhanced to a latte with non-dairy creams and sweeteners like Agave and Date syrups. 1 tsp to 6 ounces of water – use a whisk to mix in liquid.

Suggestions for coping with constipation

Constipation can accompany heavy doses of narcotic pain relievers and can be extremely painful if a stool blockage occurs, so it is important to keep bowel function at optimum level for health and comfort.

- Eat a variety of high-fiber foods
- Drink 8-10 cups of clear liquid a day
- Drink 16 ounces warm water with ½ teaspoon of Himalayan or sea salt upon rising
- Try eating every three hours daily to regulate your bowel movements.
- Limit drinks and foods that cause gas.
- Avoid drinking with a straw.
- Increase your physical activity – even leg raises while sitting in a chair helps – a walk is even better!
- Increase your fiber intake and drink fluids throughout the day to maintain hydration. Adding Psyllium flakes to drinks can aid smooth evacuation of bowels by adding much needed soft fiber to your diet.
- Medications to relieve constipation can be added at the discretion of your physician.

Suggestions for coping with Diarrhea

Diarrhea can cause severe dehydration and it is important to maintain electrolyte balance to prevent complications. It is important to eat foods containing potassium and sodium when bouts of diarrhea are experienced: potatoes, bananas, cooked vegetables, broths, saltines, and pretzels.

- Avoid drinking dairy products and foods made from milk until you feel better.
- Rest for 30 minutes after meals. Rest may slow down the digestive tract.
- Adding Psyllium flakes to drinks can aid smooth evacuation of bowels by adding much needed soft fiber to your diet.
- If you are plagued with low potassium and experience abdominal cramping or digestive pain when taking physician prescribed oral potassium, discuss this option with your physician. Organic Unsulfured Molasses is much more palatable, is equally effective, and does not cause abdominal cramping.

One tablespoon of organic Unsulfured Molasses also contains 4.5gms of iron, which means its particularly good for pregnant or menstruating women, vegetarians and people suffering from anemia. Molasses can be added to almond, coconut, or organic whole or reduced fat milk with a sweetener for cool refreshing iced drink.

Recipe - Anti-diarrhea broth

Place 2 Tablespoons white flour in a small skillet. Brown the flour slowly over medium-low heat. Be careful not to burn the flour. Once the flour is light brown add one cup of water and a bouillon packet of flavor of choice. Warm mixture on moderate heat stirring frequently until thickened. Sip slowly.

Coping with Fatigue

- Maintain light to moderate exercise each day. Short walks stimulate GI motility and appetite.

- Take naps or rest breaks often.
- Don't push yourself save your energy for activities that are most important to you.
- Avoid eating foods high in sugar. SUGAR FEEDS CANCER!
- Try eating snacks high in protein such as nuts, cottage cheese, lean poultry, tuna, salmon, peanut butter, protein shakes.
- Check with your nutritionist or naturopathic practitioner about vitamin and mineral supplements.
- Try using relaxation techniques to combat stress such as deep breathing, meditation, visualization, music therapy, or massage.
- Body toweling or body brushing helps stimulate circulation and energy.
- Take a stimulating shower by alternating hot and cold water.

Dry skin brushing improves energy levels

- Increases circulation to the skin.
- Breaks down unwanted toxins and encourages elimination of metabolic waste.
- Stimulates shedding of dead skin cells and encourages new cell growth.
- It increases circulation and lymphatic drainage.
- Stimulates the nervous system.
- It opens pores.
- Reduces fatigue.
- Strengthens the immune system
- Dry skin brushing can be done with a soft bristle brush or a

towel.
- Always dry brush before bathing.
- Brush from feet to neck because most of the lymph in your body drains to a central area near your neck.
- The entire body should be brushed including your back.
- Use light pressure in areas where the skin is thin and harder pressure on places like the soles of the feet.
- Skin brushing should be performed once a day.
- Brush in a circular motion.
- Brush upwards on the back and down from the neck.
- Have a friend, spouse or family member brush for you. It is extremely relaxing and can be used to reduce stress as well.

Suggestions for coping with Taste changes

- Practice good oral hygiene. Cancer treatments like chemotherapy can disrupt the balance in the mouth and irritate the taste buds. Keeping your mouth clean and healthy helps food taste better. Gently brush your teeth, gums and tongue with a soft bristled toothbrush in the morning, before and after meals, and before bedtime.
- Rinse your mouth frequently. Rinsing can help prevent infections, improve the healing of mouth sores and neutralize bad tastes in the mouth. Try rinsing with a mild solution of water, baking soda and salt before meals.
- Chew ¼ teaspoon of fennel after rinsing
- Experiment with different foods. Prepare foods that smell and taste good to you, even if the food is unfamiliar.
- Eat foods at the right temperature. Cold or chilled foods may taste better than warm or hot foods. Cold or room-

temperature foods also have less of an aroma.
- Add seasonings and spices to food to improve the flavor through the use of herbs and spices. Incorporate anti cancer spices at each meal to include garlic, ginger, turmeric, and onions, as well as lemon, mint, dill, basil, rosemary, and cinnamon to add a new element of flavor.

MEDITATION

Meditation has been used for thousands of years. Early origins were used to help deepen the understanding of sacred or mystical forces affecting life. Today meditation is used to de-stress and relax. Meditation is considered a type of mind-body complimentary part of medicine. When properly introduced into the mind and body a deep state of relaxation can be assumed and a sacred tranquil state can evoke a peaceful environment for the person. Meditation can balance the mind with the body creating a feeling of well-being. It can induce a healing effect on a sick body. It can help manage stressful states of anxiety, asthma, cancer, depression, heart disease, high blood pressure, pain, and sleep disorders.

There are many types of meditation. All meditation types have the ability to enhance a state of relaxation and inner peace if one is susceptible to the power of its effect. Lighting a scented candle, playing soft relaxing music, and sitting or lying in a comfortable place can promote a meditating atmosphere.

Prayer is the active communication with God. Prayer can be silent or an out loud conversation with the Creator. There are no rules to prayer. One can pray anywhere, anytime, about anything! You can take anything to God's table whenever you feel the need. I praise God in many ways. Sometimes I just sing my thoughts to the Lord. When I sing an amazing feeling of peace comes over my soul. Sometimes when I am alone in the house. I turn the phones off, light a scented candle, turn on relaxing music, close the drapes, and lay on my bed in the scant light emanating from the flicker of the candle. I breathe deeply several times taking in the pleasant fragrance of the candle. I whisper my praises and give thanks for the peace in my heart. I invite God to enter my thoughts and clear my mind so I may accept His will in my body. When I reach the state of relaxation I am searching for, I listen for God to talk to me through His spirit. I love meditating this way. Meditation to me is very different than prayer. I am mind-active in prayer and mind-inactive in meditation allowing God to be the active one.

- Guided meditation is the use of visualization. A person mentally imagines they are in a place of peaceful energy. I like to close my eyes and listen for the ocean to break on a sandy shore. You see, I have a deep love of for water and its motion. I imagine seeing gulls swoop down and pick up crumbs from the sandy shore. As I imagine seeing this I slow my breathing. I inhale slowly counting to seven, hold my breath for the count of seven, and exhale slowly counting to seven. This lowers the heart rate and brings with it lower stress. Any time I have the opportunity to sit near a shore whether it is an ocean or a Great Lake I close my eyes and take in the sounds. There is nothing more peaceful to my soul.
- Mindful meditation is experienced by increased awareness of surroundings and acceptance of what is near oneself. I experience the depth of my breathing and slowing of my heartbeat. If thoughts creep in, I usher them away and consciously will each limb to relax.
- Mantra meditation is when you repeat a word or group of

words to influence your body to come to a state of relaxation. In the Sikh religion one repeats Waheguru over and over while concentrating on their word for God. They free their mind of outside influence and concentrate on God or Waheguru.
- Qi gong is a Chinese relaxation technique combining meditation, relaxation, and physical movement to achieve a deep state of relaxation.
- Yoga is a series of postures and controlled breathing techniques used to promote flexibility and to calm the mind as a means to help one's body participate fully in the practice of meditation.
- Aroma therapy is a form of alternative medicine that uses volatile plant materials known as essential oils and other aromatic compounds for the purpose of altering a person's mind, mood, cognitive function, or health.
- Music therapy is the use of music to accomplish a calmness and less stressful state.
- Painting or art therapy uses the creative process of painting to improve the physical, mental and emotional well-being through the reduction of stress. I am a mixed media artist. I find when I am creating a canvas nothing can get into my mind but the creation I am working on. My stress and worries fade as I give my creativity the power of my thoughts. When I leave a canvas I am refreshed.
- Any one or combination of types of meditation can be beneficial. If one is not to your preference try another until you find a peaceful accomplishment.

FAITH AND SPIRITUALITY

In a Time magazine article, The Biology of Belief, dated Feb 12, 2009, Jeffrey Kluger delves deep into brain function and its response to prayer and spirituality. He was adamant the body and brain contain a lot of spiritual wiring and respond significantly to the exposure of faith activities and prayer. He also admitted, "... a growing body of scientific evidence suggests that faith may indeed bring us health."

I did not need a scientific study to inform me of the power of prayer, faith, and trust in God, but, I am glad to see there is scientific proof of this fact. You do not have to be religious to be spiritual. A belief in the Creator and a heartfelt acceptance of God's place in your life is significant. Adding meditation, prayer, or devotionals to your daily activities enhances the body's ability to heal the disease process within. I am a Believer. God is my Father and I believe God raised Jesus from the dead and He died for my sins.

"For it is with your heart that you believe and are justified, and it is with your mouth that you profess your faith and are saved." Romans 10:10

Many people have different feelings about life after death and cling to life for fear of death. Having faith or spiritual beliefs can help a person cope with a terminal disease. Cultural beliefs and spiritual needs vary person to person and religion to religion and can help a person to heal themselves through the active practice of faith.

The terms spirituality and religion are interchangeable but they have different meanings. Religion refers to a specific set of beliefs and practices whereby spirituality is the relationships people have with a force or power beyond the individual which helps them feel connected particularly in reference to the meaning of life. Anyone may think of themselves as spiritual or religious or both. Spirituality can affect quality of life through positive benefits:

- Decreased feelings of anxiety, depression, and anger
- Decreased feelings of loneliness
- Maintain normal blood pressure
- Help control pain, nausea, and dis-ease

Spirituality can help patients and families accept the circumstances of the illness, achieve personal growth while living after cancer as a survivor, and how to prepare for death if the disease is unstoppable. Many times faith and spirituality can give a person the courage to live or die depending on the circumstances. During times of pain and discomfort of treatments, or while feeling alone or lonely, these and other practices can help take you mentally to another place where you feel whole, connected, and at peace:

- Praying
- Meditation
- Breathing exercises
- Reading Bible or religious passages

- Repeating a Mantra
- Listening to spiritual music
- Practicing Yoga

Having faith also offers hope to those suffering from terminal illness and has been found to have a positive effect on the quality of life of cancer patients.

GRATITUDE

Gratitude you say? How can you have gratitude when you are facing a death sentence? Actually gratitude can be cultivated and can help by increasing a person's resilience in the face of a debilitating illness. It can open new opportunities and experiences if you will allow it. It can have an impact on the body's response to stress by balancing blood pressure and stress related symptoms. Gratitude can contribute to improved family dynamics during the process of accepting, living, and dying with cancer.

When distressing moments happen step away, grab your journal, and write down everything you are grateful for. Write until you feel the stress ease from your body.

Take time when family and friends visit to verbalize and exchange feelings of gratitude. Write letters to those who have impacted positively on your life and thank them. These are positive things that can in effect improve your situation and make you smile. Remember to carry God upon your face – it is contagious!

WHEN ENOUGH IS ENOUGH

The journey of cancer has many paths. To make a decision to stop treatment and say "Enough is Enough" can be the most painful decision you or a family member makes. This is a time when a great deal of understanding and support is necessary. One thing I want to reiterate about death and dying with cancer is: it is a dying family affair. Everyone has something to lose with the death of a loved one. Everyone will suffer in the loss one way or another.

Remember, you must live life your way and the decision to end treatment is yours to make. Your friends and family may offer their thoughts and they may not agree with your decision. The emotions surrounding this decision will bring death to the forefront. It will create additional stress, anger, fear, and concern to everyone involved. When resistance is met and demands are made it is important to gently reinforce your decision and explain why you have made the decision to end treatment.

Deciding to end treatment does not mean you are necessarily giving up the fight. You can be selective about what parts of treatment you want to end or you can stop all treatments if you choose. You may choose to end chemotherapy and radiation and opt for comfort measures and nutrition. It is about choosing to live your life your way.

It is important your family understands the process you used to make the decision. It may not be the path they would choose for you and it will be important for them to understand how you came to your decision. Family members usually take their own needs into consideration and not yours. They look at what they will be losing in the equation. Many times a decision to end treatment forces the grief process to surface sooner rather than later and it can be too much for some to bear.

One thing I can suggest is to take time to review all of your options regarding any change of treatment so you will be comfortable with your decision. Make your decision an educated choice rather than an emotional one. Even if you feel one choice is a better choice – understand all of the options and be prepared to answer questions friends and family will undoubtedly ask.

It is important to understand the difference between benefits of treatment and side effects. Most western treatments do not cure cancer and are given primarily to slow cancer's spread. Notice, I said most. There may be rare instances of cure or remission but they are usually accompanied with changes in lifestyle and those changes are rarely given credit for the transformation or cure of a disease process. My point is, you do not have to give up on your disease because of side effects related to your current treatment if it is showing positive shrinkage. Treat the symptoms with changes in lifestyle. However, if you are showing no change in cancer growth and side effects are disallowing quality of life then by all means feel comfortable in stopping or changing you current treatment.

Active faith and spirituality can be beneficial as you make this decision through approaching this time in your life without a fear of dying. Seek comfort through prayer for strength as you make this decision and have faith in the afterlife God promises.

It is important to reinforce with family and friends stopping treatment does not mean you are giving up on the disease or on living. It means you are taking responsibility for your quality of life. Never apologize for making a decision regarding your comfort or care.

I made some very uncomfortable decisions regarding my life and the life of my parents. I made the choice to ignore western philosophy and medicine and made a change in lifestyle regarding my own care. When it came to my parents the decision was extremely difficult.

My father had been in a comatose state for many months and was being fed by tube for bodily nourishment and given total care by a nursing home staff. He had wasted from an upright 150 pounds to 88 pounds of emaciated body mass twisted into a fetal position. When my father developed a high fever I consulted a physician and friend of mine regarding discontinuation of treatment.

My concern was, if I withheld life sustaining care would my father suffer pain and in his state of illness may not be able to convey his pain. My friend assured me my father would suffer no pain by the withholding of nourishment. He explained the body's response and how even when conscious the feeling of hunger was rare in this point of the disease process.

I made the decision to stop the feedings and decline further treatment and life support. I was criticized by the nursing home staff and even told I was being cruel. I took it hard as I prayed for God's forgiveness for my choice but I knew it was necessary and the right decision. My father died the day following the discontinuation of care – and I was at his side.

Six weeks later I was faced with a decision regarding my mother's care. She had been in a coma for three weeks and had suffered a fractured spine when turned by the nursing staff. This was not an injury caused by mishandling. It was related to the cancerous state of metastatic disease to the bone. My mother had also developed a cease of activity in the intestines related to the fracture, swelling of the spinal cord, and an infarct in the vessels leading to the bowel. It was only a matter of time she would have gangrene and a raging untreatable sepsis causing more damage.

A decision had to be made and I chose to allow placement of an intravenous of pain medication to allow total comfort for my mother. My mother died within two hours of the administration of the medication.

I admit I felt terrible grief and guilt following my decisions in both circumstances and somehow felt as though I took precious moments from my parent's lives when in reality I loved them enough to allow them the peace of death. It took time for me to accept this but I am comfortable today with my decisions.

Nutrition and End of Life

How much someone nearing the end of life needs nutritionally can be an enigma. Family members feel helpless to help their loved one and often food is the only avenue they know to show their love for the individual, but, at end of life food is generally the last thing a cancer patient needs. Caregivers and family members need to be aware a normal part of the dying process is for organs to shut down. Pushing fluids and food at this time can cause more harm than good. Nutrition should be offered in the form of broths and smoothies more for hydration than nutritional value and they need to be aware an overload of fluid in the body can also cause the patient to be very uncomfortable. Most cancer patients are not hungry near the end of life. Their major need is comfort and pain relief.

Feeding through a feeding tube should be related to nutritional needs primarily to provide strength and improve quality of life. If the patient has a chance for recovery and is suffering loss of appetite I agree with an enteral feeding, but, if it is end of life and the patient can no longer tolerate food I pray family members will show love and compassion for their loved one and allow them to be free of the complications associated with feeding at the end of life such as intolerance of feeding, nausea, vomiting, and severe diarrhea. It is not easy to love someone enough to honor their wishes and withhold life saving nutrition.

Planning for Death - Legal Affairs

There is an emergence of a new advocacy in patient care as laws and/or a person's personal wishes for care are not being enforced by hospitals and/or care providers. A patient advocate is an individual who typically acts as liaison between a patient and their health care provider. Generally they have a professional background. Often they have been case managers in the field of social work or are nurses. They know how to navigate the bureaucracy of large health plans and are trained professionals who have re-focused on helping patients in their decision-making, coordination of care, and seeing their wishes are followed.

Addressing your legal and financial affairs is very important and must be done as soon as possible following your diagnosis. Having peace of mind and knowing your wishes will be followed is paramount to your healing process. You can specify how everything you own is to be distributed after your death. You can legalize your personal wishes for; medical care, and whom you will entrust medical decision making in the event of your incapacitation and appoint a person who will be your voice should you be unable to communicate. You can gain peace of mind knowing you have done your best to protect what you want done and relieve your family of the stress of trying to make decisions.

A Living Will or Healthcare Directive

A Living Will or Healthcare Directive is a legal form where you can document your personal health care directions regarding heroic care. It will inform medical personnel whether you want to be resuscitated in the event your heart stops, whether you want to be placed on a breathing machine if you stop breathing, whether you want to be fed with a feeding tube if you are unable to eat. It contains your personal directions for your care. It is important to note: Hospitals do not always feel legally bound by a Living Will. State laws vary and all it takes is a family member insisting on specific care and the hospital does not follow your wishes. It is important your loved ones know where you stand on all issues. Take note: This document is only used if you become incapacitated. You personally can revoke this document at any time as long as you are able to make competent decisions.

Durable Power of Attorney (POA) for health

Durable Power of Attorney (POA) for health care allows another person legal rights to make decisions for you as your health care proxy in the event you are unable to do it for yourself.

Choose a trusted family member, a close friend, or a legal advocate such as an attorney. Be sure to ask if they are willing to be your POA. It is important you have a lengthy discussion with the person you choose. You must share what you expect from them regarding your care. Make sure they know every detail listed on your Living Will and where to find it. It is best to give them a legal copy to keep with them. This legal document must be signed in front of a notary public to be legal.

Durable Power of Attorney for Finance

Durable Power of Attorney for Finance gives the named person the legal authority to act on your behalf with regard to your finances temporarily. They can take care of your banking and pay your bills as long as you are incapacitated. When you are able to resume your personal business the power is returned to you. You can choose the same person you name as POA of health care or someone else you trust your finances with.

Wills and Estate Planning

Wills and Estate planning should be addressed with an Attorney. This is one legal form of utmost importance. This form allows you to specify where and who will receive your assets in the event of your death. A will even determines the custody of your children and who will assume their care and how your assets will be used to support their care. An attorney will guide you through the many choices you have. Even though there are online forms with instructions and do-it-yourself forms an attorney knows everything you will need to cover in a will. One mistake can keep an estate in limbo for years.

Note: You can download copies of these documents from the website lordimnotdoneyet.com. All legal documents must be signed in front of a notary public to be legal. Until that time they will not be valid or honored by medical establishments. You can also download Advanced Directives by selecting your state at http://www.caringinfo.org/i4a/pages/index.cfm?pageid=3289

Advance Funeral Arrangements

Advance funeral arrangements assure your wishes will be

honored. Advanced planning saves your family from having to make decisions when they are in a state of grief. Advance planning can include buying of burial plots, space in a mausoleum, or arrangements for cremation. Each type carries a different price and funeral homes are required by law to reveal item by item cost.

Palliative Care

Palliative care focuses on medical treatment of pain or slowing of disease process rather than providing a cure. This is usually provided in a hospital or nursing home. The goals of palliative care includes: comfort, quality of life needs, and spiritual needs.

Hospice Care

Hospice care is a specific kind of end of life care. It is limited to the last six months of life, (time deemed by physician,) and is offered 24 hours a day in the dying person's home. The focus of Hospice is to provide pain management, medical care, spiritual and emotional support for the patient and their family members. Hospice leads everyone through the death, dying, and grief process. I have noticed an increase of Hospice care facilities cropping up as the need for this type of care increases. Many families are fearful of having a family member die at home.

Making Decisions about Your Funeral

Making decisions about your funeral may not be something you want to address, but, through advanced planning and making your wishes known, you can relieve your loved ones from the task while they are grieving and in pain over your loss.

Many times families cannot make decisions following the loss of a loved one. Disagreements arise with personal circumstances influencing those involved. While one family member may consider limiting unnecessary costs in an attempt to contain expenses another may be drawn to provide the very best offered in a last ditch effort to show their undying love for an individual without thinking of where the money will come from to pay for the decisions they make. There are funeral homes who will suggest top of the line items taking full advantage of a grieving family. It assures those types of funeral directors great profit. It is important to research and select a reputable funeral home. Your family will be grateful they do not have to address this.

This is a very good reason to make advanced funeral arrangements. It relieves your loved ones from the responsibility and gives the person making the arrangements a peace of mind knowing it will be carried out their way.

Advanced planning can include but is not necessarily limited to buying a burial plot, mausoleum, or deciding to be cremated. The costs are remarkably different but the decision will be a matter of your personal preference.

Be aware: funeral homes charge for everything including but not limited to caskets, vaults, religious services, ceremonies, transportation, viewing hours, personnel, arrangement of offerings of respect, embalming, and body preparation (make-up, hair, clothing application.) Additional charges will be incurred by the cemetery or mausoleum, opening of grave site or mausoleum drawer, and sealing of same, placement of vault and lowering devices, preparation for service at site, and personnel. Many of these expenses are required and must be paid for in advance.

Advanced planning can be a family project or a personal one. Advance planning can be arranged and paid for over time. Shopping around can greatly influence the price of funeral arrangements. Advanced planning gives you more time to consider your options and make informed decisions without feeling rushed into making decisions. You will feel a sense of peace knowing arrangements are completed and your family will be free of last minute details.

Pre-payment allows you to lock into today's prices. Some funeral homes have financing available for pre planning, or you can seek financing through an institution of your choice. By prepaying your estate will not incur the debt of your funeral.

Funerals are touted as the traditional way to recognize the finality of death and are rituals for the living to show their respect for the dead. It is also recognized to help survivors begin the grieving process.

The minute someone dies and the message of death is received the death is real. Yes, we may wish it was not so, but, we know in our heart of hearts it has happened. I did not need to see my mother's body in a casket in a funeral home to feel the pain of loss in my heart, but, there are some who cannot accept a death as real without observing the body in its final state.

My ideal plan is to be cremated. Although viewing is a part of many cultural and ethnic traditions I do not feel the need to have a viewing. The time I have spent with others while I am alive is what is important to me and a celebration of life in a place chosen by my family is my desire. I want my family and friends to gather for a meal a few weeks after my passing and celebrate not grieve. I want them to know I am in a place chosen by God and I am accepting of my passing.

I have known for as long as I have had memory, we are all born with a time to die. I have had my bags packed for many years. I have no fear of the hereafter. I will embrace it with an open heart.

Mourning and Grief

The stages of mourning and grief are universal and are experienced by everyone who has had a loss or a catastrophic event in their lives, including the diagnosis of a life threatening disease process or illness. There are five stages of normal grief that were first proposed by Elisabeth Kübler-Ross in her 1969 book "On Death and Dying."

In the process of mourning, a different length of time is spent working through each step and each stage can be more or less intense. The five stages do not necessarily occur in order and one often moves between stages before reaching a peaceful acceptance of the loss or impending death. Many times one is not afforded the luxury of time required to achieve the final stage of grief. The disease process ends their lives prematurely and they die in a mixed stage of fear and acceptance.

Impending death leads us to reevaluate our life, its longevity, and our mortality. We tend to move our mind over the time wasted in our lives, a time when we did nothing, a time we could have spent doing something important, but, did not. It is time lost forever. It then can overwhelm our thinking about, "What have I done?"

Many people will not experience the grieving process in the same way and not everyone will go through all of the stages of grief. Kübler-Ross was adamant about this point when she detailed the process of grief. To understand the stages is not to feel like you must go through each one of them in order. Instead, it is more important to look at them as a guide in the grieving process. It will help you understand and put into context where you are in the grieving process.

Kübler-Ross Stages of Grief

Stage I - Denial and Isolation

The first reaction to learning of terminal illness or impending death is to deny the reality of the situation. It is a normal reaction to rationalize your emotions. Rationalization is a defense mechanism that buffers the immediate shock. You may block out the words and hide from the facts. This is a temporary response that will carry you through the first wave of pain.

Stage II - Anger

As denial and isolation begins to take its toll on your well being, reality and its pain re-emerge. Intense emotion will attack your vulnerable core. This emotion is expressed as anger. The anger may be directed at family, friends, complete strangers, and even God as you process the devastating emotions consuming your consciousness. Anger may be directed at the one you love the most. You know the person is not to blame but in some way may resent you are being forced to live with a decision in which we had no part in making. You may feel guilty for being angry, and this may even make you angrier.

Stage III - Bargaining

The third stage involves the hope that one can somehow postpone or delay death. A negotiation for an extension of life is made with a higher power in exchange for a promise to change the way one lives. The helplessness and vulnerability consumes one's thoughts of a way to stop the horrific disease process within them – thus allowing them more time. One may bargain if only I had sought medical attention sooner if only I had not smoked, if only I been a better person, if only I had gone to church, if only I had given more to the needy, if only... if only.

Stage IV - Depression

During the fourth stage one begins to understand the certainty of death. It is not acceptance but knowledge of death being imminent. The individual may become silent, refuse visitors and spend most of the time crying and isolating themselves from others. This allows one to extract themselves from love and affection which stimulates reality. It is an important time in the grieving process. It's natural to feel sadness, regret, fear, and uncertainty when going through this stage. Feeling these emotions show one has begun to accept the situation. Not that they agree with the ill health but understand the process they are experiencing.

Stage V - Acceptance

In this last stage, individuals begin to come to terms with their mortality and not everyone reaches this stage. Death may be sudden and unexpected or one may never see beyond their anger or denial stage.

This stage is also a negative stage of grief but is not the same as depression. This stage may find one withdrawn, quiet, and calm beyond understanding by family and friends. Ones dignity and grace maybe the last gift we give to our loved ones.

Going through the grieving process is a deeply personal experience and no one can help us through it. Sometimes the good will offered by others becomes an intrusion on our acceptance or denial of our illness. No one can understand the emotions you are feeling or the fear consuming your inner being. It is important to allow yourself to feel the grief as it comes over you. Resisting it only will prolong the natural process of healing.

FOOD FOR THOUGHT - MY FINAL WORDS

Through my life I have been influenced by people I have been exposed to, but, more importantly by the many ideas I have read, words I have heard spoken, and images I have seen. Some of these experiences leave my thoughts as soon as my senses move to experience something new. I opened myself to subjects I never had interest in and learned so many valuable points of view I would have otherwise remained ignorant about. The most important and influential things I learned were those affecting my spirituality and philosophical view; those that touched my heart and soul.

I am philosophical in my own right and when I am influenced by another view. To me it has to be an amazing view, because I am not easily swayed from my way of thinking. I love a good debate but hate arguments. Debates give us an opportunity to lay out our beliefs and hear someone else's. Arguments close our minds to what others are saying.

I might ask, do you have a point in your life when all was well, a time when everything was good, and in your memory you can immediately find a place in time you felt safe and warm and at peace, a time when you were less stressed, happier, and very content? Can you think about that time and compare it to your way of living at this moment and think about the differences from then to now. Age and health status aside what has changed? Let's go through what I perceive as the top things which could have changed in your life.

I imagine relationships may be one of the top contenders. Maybe you are alone, have always been alone, are divorced, or are dealing with a difficult relationship, or have recently broken a relationship which meant a lot to you. A warm, nurturing relationship makes up a large part of life. When facing a terminal illness alone it can be devastating. If you are alone try to change this aspect of your life. There are cancer support groups in most communities. For additional support get involved in a church community and it does not have to be one of your particular faith. Go online and research the churches in your area. Most churches have websites and list their monthly activities. You can call any church and ask to meet the pastor. Pastors love introducing new attendees to the congregation and most congregations have open arms for new worshipers. For recreational events join a Meet Up group. There are many activities planned and posted for anyone to attend near most communities at http://www.meetup.com/.

Financial situations change throughout our lives. Maybe you need more income or hate your job, or your job is more demanding of your time than you like. Do your best to downsize your living arrangements if this is the issue. If the financial need is related to healthcare, contact a local hospital and ask to speak to a social worker and ask for a list of community services which offer help to those in need.

Are you too worrisome and it affects the wellbeing of your mental and physical environment? Worry can literally stop you in your tracks. It requires great energy to worry and will deplete your entire store of energy in one sitting. It creates a negative atmosphere and with it comes depression. My cure all for worry is to give my worries to God. I have a God Can, a cardboard can, I have decorated with material and nice trinkets and a placard that says "GOD CAN." I have a stack of 4"x4" papers nearby. When I feel worried or have something to give to God, I write it on one of the papers and place it in the can giving it to Him. I tell God this is for Him to carry for me because I have no room to deal with it nor the energy to waste on it. Three to six months later I empty the can and read what I gave to God. I am amazed when I read and realize how the problem or worry that influenced my heart so much had been dealt with and without my input.

Are you a control freak? Do you feel the need to have absolute control over everything in your life? Realize right now, no one is capable of controlling anything but themselves and even that can be difficult when subconscious thoughts take over! My best friend has OCD, Obsessive Compulsive Disorder, at least I tell him that. He has a need to over think every detail of something ten times over and then some. He has an extremely analytical mind and occupation. It drives him crazy and inadvertently me as well, because he constantly asks my opinion and then he obsesses over my opinion ten times over and then some. It is a repetitive action and sometimes we make gentle headway but more often than not he continues to try to control everything. To be at peace one must realize there is no controlling life. We can influence it. Everyone must realize, in the end to all ends, life controls us and God controls life.

Do you live your life comparing yourself to others? Are you in the mindset of, "Keeping up with the Joneses?" Not familiar with that term? "Keeping up with the Joneses" is an idiom in the English language about how someone compares themselves to their neighbor in relationship to an accumulation of material things. In illness, it is important not to compare yourself to others. The doctors may use statistics to explain treatment options, but, not everyone is the same. You have a completely unique set of circumstances. Yes, you may have a specific strain of cancer but your circumstances will be completely different than a person in your community with the same strain of cancer. So "keeping up with the Joneses" is an unacceptable option. Treatment choices and their effectiveness are all about you and how your individual body responds no matter how many statistics are out there.

Are you constantly reliving your past? Feeling guilty? Having regrets? Terminal illness tends to bring these feelings to the forefront as we ponder the "why" of it. The thought of what did I do wrong can be devastating. You cannot relive the past but if you made mistakes that can be reversed by all means make an attempt to reverse those causes. Otherwise leave it all behind. Living the past adds burdens and drains energy. We need the energy to heal ourselves. Don't sabotage your energy levels this way.

Are you a procrastinator? I am. I will put something off to the last second sometimes and then kick myself over my stupidity! Terminal illness will not stand for procrastination. The changes necessary for healing must be moved upon immediately. Delaying in this can only mean failure and death.

Are you afraid of dying? You could be afraid of the probability of timing of death but the actual act of death should never be feared if you are a believer. God is your Father and He has prepared a place for you. I have been there. I know it exists. Do not fear the afterlife. It is a place free of pain and worry where there is a joining of community as none here on earth.

Do you know God? Do you have faith, spirituality, a belief there is a Creator? Being with others who share your beliefs and teachings can fulfill emotional needs and improve well being. It can add to your mental outlook regarding your disease and the path it takes.

Have you not learned from your mistakes? Do you smoke even though you have lung cancer? Do you consume alcohol even though you have pancreatic cancer? In order to learn from your mistakes you must take ownership of them and make a commitment to change this behavior. Realize your mistakes have helped bring you to this disease process.

I have shared many ideas within the pages of this book. My heart and soul believes you have the power to heal yourself by the grace of God. Take charge of your destiny. Never allow anyone to bully you into doing something you do not want to do and most of all, Live your life your way.

"Lord I'm not done yet!" ~

Invite Phyllis to Speak to Your Group, Organization, or Congregation

Phyllis has a dynamic, engaging personality, and has a way of drawing her audience into active participation to improve upon their lifestyle weaknesses as they face the diagnosis of cancer. She is passionate about helping others find the inner strength to live life their way and connect with a spiritual peace in accepting, living, and dying with cancer.

She takes her audience on a positive journey as she shares her personal story of and how she chose to take a non-traditional path to healing when it was virtually unheard of. She has been known to bring audiences to tears as she challenges them to take charge of their destiny.

What stands out about her presentations above all else is her generosity of heart and her belief in God's power to heal a disease even when the medical profession says it can't be done.

She is a Believer and when time allows she lays hands on and prays with conference attendees leaving them uplifted, inspired, and armed to fight their battle with confidence.

Join the Lord I'm Not Done Yet community at phyllislomaxsingh.com or lordimnotdoneyet.com

If you would like to:
- Schedule an online appointment
- Book a speaking engagement
- Arrange a book signing event
- Follow the LINDY blog
- Post questions
- Seek a referral
- Seek Prayer or Healing Hands
- Find recipes for a healthy fit lifestyle
- Order a LINDY Journal
- Order a LINDY bracelet
- Order a LINDY book marker
- Order a LINDY Medical Planner

Follow on twitter: Phyllis Lomax Singh

Join the LINDY Facebook page: Lord I'm Not Done Yet

Reference page

Advanced Directives by State

http://www.caringinfo.org/i4a/pages/index.cfm?pageid=3289

American Cancer Society

http://www.cancer.org/

Andrew Weil, MD

Director of the Center for Integrative Medicine of the College of Medicine, University of Arizona

http://www.drweilblog.com

http://www.drweil.com/

Angiogenesis Foundation diet

http://www.eattobeat.org/

Association of Cancer Online Resources

http://www.acor.org

Cancer Centers of America

http://www.cancercenter.com

Community Meet up

http://www.meetup.com/

Francois Theberge, MD, CHHC

CEO @ The Health of the Matter

mindful@healthofthematter.com

Go green products

http://www.greenhome.com/

Go green newsletter

http://www2.epa.gov/newsroom/gogreen

Hippocrates Health Institute

http://hippocratesinst.org/

Dr Li's Ted Talk

https://www.ted.com/talks/william_li

She is our Mother

She is the whisper of a breeze that rustles leaves as you walk down a path.
She is the wind who bends trees to splitting in a tornado.
She is the ice crystals forming on a window pane in the frigid cold.
She is the fragrance of flowers carried through an open window as they bloom.
She is the heat of the sun and the cool mist of a fog.
She is the rat-a-tat-tat of rain that lull's you to sleep on a stormy night or the clap of thunder which startles you awake.
She is the salt in the ocean and clouds in the sky.
She is the cool refreshing water running from a crevice in a rock.
She is the soil from which our plants grow.
She is precious. She is nature.
She needs replenished and protected.
She is our Mother - Our Mother Earth.

LORD I'M NOT DONE YET

Phyllis Lomax Singh

ALPHABETICAL INDEX

Acceptance 59, 85, 111, 115, 135, 137, 150, 152
Acupuncture 16
Advocate 144, 145
Afterlife 112, 141, 156
Agave 126, 127, 128
Airborne 36
Alcohol 156
Allergies 30
Allopathic 9
Alpha-lipoic 55
Alternative 8, 15, 17, 61, 117, 136
Aluminum 32
Amines 19
Amino 42, 128
Anemia 13, 46, 56, 130
Anger 69, 80, 104, 138, 140, 151, 152
Angiogenesis 20, 21, 22, 23, 119, 160
Angiogenesis-based 22
Anti-angiogenesis 15, 21, 23
Anti-angiogenic 20, 22
Anti-cancer 20, 49, 50, 118, 119
Anti-diarrhea 130
Anti-inflammatory 49, 50, 52
Anti-nausea 120
Antineoplastic 117
Antioxidant 48, 50, 52, 118, 128
Antioxidants 49, 52, 54, 119, 120, 128
Antiseptic 119
Anxiety 2, 6, 45, 56, 62, 80, 85, 134, 138
Appetite 44, 45, 72, 73, 130, 144
Appointment 11, 70, 84, 159
Arguments 153
Art 67, 136
Arthritis 18, 118
Aspirin 55
Asthma 134
Asthmatics 30
Atherosclerosis 18
Attorney 6, 145, 146
Ayurveda 15, 118
Ayurvedic 16, 117, 118
Bacteria 26, 29, 32, 33, 34, 119, 122
Baldness 13
Bargain 106, 107, 151
Bath 26, 120, 121, 132
Bedfast 78, 102
Behavior 16, 73, 74, 77, 85, 157
Belief 15, 113, 137, 156, 158
Beliefs 58, 67, 101, 137, 138, 153, 156
Believe 37, 56, 60, 64, 67, 75, 91, 107, 112, 113, 115, 137
Believer 27, 86, 102, 105, 113, 114, 115, 137, 156, 158
Bible 113, 138
Bile 109, 121, 122, 123
Biliary 109, 110
Biofeedback 16
Bisphenol 31
Bladder 122, 123
Blame 87, 95, 151
Blessed 8, 64, 94, 98
Blessings 2, 113, 114, 115
Blood 5, 13, 20, 21, 27, 38, 40, 41, 46, 51, 103, 110, 117, 119, 128, 134, 138, 139
Blood-forming 5
Botanicals 16
Boundaries 85
Bowel 18, 37, 46, 54, 122, 123, 129, 130, 143
Brain 6, 16, 27, 37, 77, 103, 137
Breast 27, 50, 51, 52, 53, 77, 104, 105, 107, 108, 114, 115, 118
Brew 48, 119, 127, 128
Brewing 17, 48, 127, 128
Broths 47, 125, 129, 130, 143
Brushing 131, 132
Bullied 5, 10
Burial 64, 147, 148
Calcium 54
Cancer 1, 2, 5, 6, 7, 8, 9, 10, 11, 12, 13, 14, 15, 16, 17, 18, 19, 20, 21, 22, 23, 27, 28, 40, 41, 44, 45, 46, 48, 49, 50, 51, 52, 53, 56, 59, 66, 69, 70, 71, 72, 76, 77, 80, 81, 82, 83, 84, 85, 93, 101, 102, 106, 108, 109, 118, 119, 120, 123, 125, 128, 131, 132, 133, 134, 138, 139, 140, 141, 143, 154, 155, 156, 157, 158, 160, 161
Cancerous 12, 19, 105, 118, 119, 142
Cancers 6, 19, 20, 27, 50, 51, 52
Canola 39
Carbohydrate 40, 41, 42, 47, 51
Carbon 29
Carcinogenic 19
Carcinogens 29, 30, 31
Carcinoma 5
Cardamom 46, 125, 126, 127, 128
Cardiovascular 40, 48, 128
Caregiver 28, 77, 81, 102, 143
Carotenoids 52, 54
Carpet 30
Catastrophic 150
Catechins 48, 119
Celiac 18
Charred 19, 29
Chemicals 7, 24, 25, 26, 28, 30, 31, 32, 33, 34, 37, 50, 119
Chemo 13, 48, 125
Chemotherapeutic 16, 21
Chemotherapy 7, 8, 10, 11, 12, 13, 44, 56, 73, 105, 119, 123, 132, 140
Chew 121, 125, 132
Chiropractic 16
Chlorine 7, 29
Cholesterol 40, 42, 119, 128
Christ 86, 112
Chromium 119
Chronic 17, 18, 56, 122
Church 101, 151, 154
Circulation 30, 38, 75, 131
Clean 7, 24, 28, 29, 30, 74, 109, 132
Cleaning 24, 30, 31, 34, 119
Cleanses 117, 122,123
Clergy 2
Climate 38
Cling-wrapped 32

164

Clinicians 10, 46
Coach 8, 10, 46, 65, 114, 115
Coenzyme 55
Colitis 122
Colon 49, 52, 122, 123
Colonic 121, 122, 123
Colorectal 19, 51
Comfort 69, 83, 86, 90, 102, 103, 129, 140, 141, 142, 143, 147
Communicate 82, 84, 85, 91, 92, 111, 144
Communication 42, 65, 70, 71, 76, 81, 82, 85, 98, 134
Community 24, 25, 27, 82, 111, 154, 156, 158, 161
Compassion 14, 80, 111, 144
Constipation 45, 46, 47, 53, 122, 123, 129
Containers 24, 25, 29, 31, 32, 33, 37, 53
Containing 25, 47, 55, 129
Contains 118, 119, 130, 145
Cookware 34
COPD 18
Cope 1, 2, 5, 81, 82, 85, 138
Cosmetics 34
Craving 48
Creator 86, 102, 113, 134, 137, 156
Cremation 147
Crohn's 122
D-alpha-tocopherol 54
Darjeeling 128
De-stress 67, 69, 134
Dead 96, 103, 121, 131, 137, 149
Death 6, 10, 14, 36, 64, 73, 77, 78, 81, 83, 96, 101, 103, 104, 106, 109, 111, 137, 138, 139, 140, 143, 144, 146, 147, 149, 150, 151, 152, 156
Debate 153
Debilitating 87, 101, 139
Deficiencies 118, 120
Dehydration 125, 129
Designated 82, 123
Detoxification 20, 117, 119, 120, 121, 122, 123
Detoxing 38
Diabetes 117
Diagnosed 27, 28, 72, 77, 80, 118
Diagnosis 1, 2, 5, 6, 9, 10, 12, 13, 15, 20, 27, 44, 59, 76, 77, 80, 81, 82, 83, 85, 93, 101, 144, 150, 158
Diarrhea 38, 45, 46, 129, 144
Diary 68
Die 1, 76, 81, 89, 111, 138, 147, 149, 150
Died 27, 78, 137, 142, 143
Diet 10, 15, 17, 18, 20, 24, 38, 39, 40, 42, 44, 46, 48, 49, 51, 54, 60, 108, 122, 129, 130, 160
Dietary 23, 44, 54, 55, 56, 61, 63, 108, 123, 125
Dietitian 10, 46
Digest 6, 50, 105, 106
Digestion 18, 36, 41, 42, 121, 122, 123
Digestive 13, 51, 121, 122, 130
Digests 36
Dignity 152
Directives 145, 146, 160
Dis-ease 59, 62, 69, 71, 138
Disability 18
Disagreement 71, 91, 92
Discomfort 61, 138
Discontinuation 83, 117, 142
Disease 6, 8, 9, 14, 17, 18, 19, 21, 36, 40, 41, 48, 59, 68, 69, 71, 76, 80, 81, 86, 101, 106, 118, 122, 128, 134, 137, 138, 141, 142, 147, 150, 151, 156, 157, 158
Disorders 18, 56, 134, 155
Doctor 10, 12, 14, 55, 61, 96, 103, 104, 106, 107, 108
Doctors 6, 10, 14, 98, 118, 155
Download 146
Downsize 154
Dreams 58, 66, 68
Drink 33, 37, 46, 47, 53, 54, 120, 122, 123, 124, 127, 129, 130
Drugs 13, 62, 73
Dr Weil 19, 55, 160
Dry-clean 30
Dust 30
Dying 80, 83, 102, 139, 140, 141, 143, 147, 150, 156, 158
Dysfunction 13, 36, 56
Ease 59, 64, 121, 139
Eco-friendly 30
EGCg 119
Electrolyte 38, 129
Electromagnetic 16
Elimination 36, 53, 122, 131
Emotional 57, 63, 64, 65, 82, 87, 102, 136, 141, 147, 151, 156
Emotions 9, 60, 64, 65, 71, 80, 140, 151, 152
Empower 44, 45, 59, 60, 74
Enable 22
Endocrine 31
Endometrial 52
Endostatin 50
Enema 122
Energy 7, 10, 16, 26, 36, 38, 39, 42, 45, 46, 56, 57, 61, 72, 73, 74, 87, 104, 114, 131, 135, 154, 155, 156
Enteral 144
Environment 7, 14, 24, 25, 27, 28, 30, 31, 37, 46, 56, 61, 63, 64, 80, 88, 118, 134, 154
Environmentally 33
Environmentally-friendly 31
Epa 28, 34, 55, 161
Esophagus 118
Estate 146, 149
Eternity 100
Exfoliation 121
Faith 1, 2, 8, 10, 68, 69, 86, 99, 101, 102, 105, 107, 112, 113, 116, 137, 138, 139, 141, 154, 156
Families 7, 18, 25, 82, 83, 103, 138, 147, 148
Family 2, 6, 11, 27, 29, 58, 66, 67, 69, 71, 72, 73, 80, 81, 82, 83, 84, 85, 86, 87, 91, 92, 95, 99, 101, 103, 132, 139, 140, 141, 143, 144, 145, 147, 148, 149, 151, 152
Fatigue 18, 38, 45, 46, 72, 73, 120, 130, 131
Fats 39, 40, 42, 50
Fear 2, 6, 57, 84, 85, 88, 89, 91, 111, 114, 137, 140, 141, 149, 150, 152, 156
Feared 21, 156
Fearful 97, 147
Fences 91, 95
Fiber 38, 41, 42, 46, 47, 51, 53, 119, 129, 130
Fibromyalgia 18
Filtration 37
Finances 63, 146, 149
Financial 6, 58, 76, 88, 144, 154
Flavanoids 48, 52
Fluoridated 7

Folate 42, 52
Folic 50, 51, 54
Forgiveness 89, 90, 102, 142
Formaldehyde 34
Forms 39, 48, 118, 146
Fructose 41
Funerals 149
Garlic 22, 49, 118, 133
Genetic 19, 36
Ginger 46, 49, 55, 119, 120, 125, 128, 133
Ginseng 22
Glioma 27
Glucose 41, 42, 51
Glycemic 51, 52
Glycemic-load 51
GMOs 7, 29, 119
Goals 21, 59, 66, 68, 69, 83, 147
God 8, 10, 57, 60, 64, 68, 69, 75, 78, 86, 90, 94, 96, 98, 99, 100, 102, 104, 105, 106, 107, 111, 112, 113, 114, 115, 116, 134, 135, 136, 137, 139, 141, 149, 151, 154, 155, 156, 157
Gods 113
God's 96, 104, 111, 113, 114, 115, 116, 134, 137, 142, 158
Go green 28, 161
Green 22, 28, 30, 31, 48, 52, 119, 127, 128, 161
Green home 28, 161
Grief 141, 143, 147, 150, 151, 152
Grieve 149
Grieving 85, 147, 148, 149, 150, 152
Grill 19, 40
Guilt 81, 83, 87, 143
Guilty 69, 151, 156
Healer 114
Healing 6, 7, 8, 10, 16, 17, 19, 20, 21, 24, 44, 46, 56, 59, 60, 61, 63, 64, 68, 69, 71, 75, 80, 81, 87, 89, 92, 101, 102, 113, 114, 115, 116, 118, 119, 132, 134, 144, 152, 156, 158, 159
Health 7, 8, 10, 11, 15, 16, 17, 19, 24, 29, 31, 36, 40, 45, 46, 48, 53, 59, 60, 61, 63, 64, 66, 69, 104, 115, 118, 124, 129, 136, 137, 144, 145, 146, 152, 153, 161
Healthcare 8, 145, 154
Healthy 7, 15, 17, 24, 25, 36,
40, 41, 42, 45, 46, 47, 48, 49, 50, 51, 52, 56, 59, 64, 66, 67, 80, 83, 102, 120, 132, 159
Heaven 90, 104, 112
Herbal 14, 16, 117, 118, 122, 123
Herbicides 7
Herbs 15, 49, 60, 133
Hereafter 149
Hereditary 18
Heritage 24, 25
Heterocyclic 19
High-fiber 129
High-quality 127
Higher 128, 151
Hippocrates 161
Hodgkin's 27
Holistic 2, 7, 8, 9, 10, 16, 20, 21, 24, 46, 59, 61, 63, 64, 115
Holistically 21, 23, 62
Homeopathy 16
Hope 2, 10, 68, 139, 151
Hopefulness 2
Hopeless 72
Hopelessness 73, 80
Hormones 39, 75
Hospice 147
Hydrating 47
Hydration 37, 46, 129, 143
Hydrogen 26, 32
Hydrogenated 40
Hygiene 132
Immune 6, 18, 20, 34, 131
Immunity 16, 45
Indian 15, 118, 128
Infection 45, 110
Infections 132
Inflammation 17, 18, 48, 49, 51, 118, 121
Inflammatory 14, 17, 18, 20, 41, 48, 49, 56, 61, 69
Inspirational 74
Insulin 42, 119
Intestines 118, 121, 122, 123, 143
Isoflavones 50
Isolation 151
Jealousy 69
Job 37, 62, 103, 110, 154
Joints 37, 53
Joneses 155, 156
Journal 11, 50, 67, 68, 69, 139, 159
Journaling 67, 68
Joys 67
Judge 90
Judgment 92
Kidney 51
Kolhoff 88
Kubler-ross 150, 151
Lactose 41
Legal 144, 145, 146
Legalize 144, 145
Letters 33, 69, 94, 95, 99, 139
Leukemia 5, 27
Lifestyle 6, 8, 10, 14, 17, 46, 59, 61, 63, 66, 80, 83, 141, 142, 158, 159
Lipids 39
Loneliness 138
Loss 8, 45, 57, 67, 73, 81, 90, 120, 140, 144, 147, 148, 149, 150
Low-glycemic-load 51
Lung 27, 52, 118, 156
Lupus 18
Lycopene 53
Lymph 5, 104, 107, 132
Lymphatic 131
Lymphocytic 27
Lymphoma 6, 27
Machta 128
Magnesium 42, 50, 51, 119
Make-up 148
Malignant 5, 12
Mammogram 103, 107
Mangosteen 120
Mantra 135, 139
Ma.riage 102
Married 27, 80, 95
Massage 16, 61, 78, 131
Matcha 48, 119, 125, 128
Mausoleum 147, 148
Meal 47, 49, 54, 55, 133, 149
Meals 19, 46, 47, 51, 57, 125, 130, 132
Mealtime 47
Meats 19, 39, 42, 49
Medication 61, 110, 117, 143
Medications 13, 21, 62, 110, 117, 120, 126, 129
Medicine 15, 16, 19, 21, 22, 24, 78, 120, 123, 134, 136, 142, 160
Meditating 134, 135
Meditation 15, 16, 62, 75, 114, 115, 131, 134, 135, 136, 137, 138
Meetup 154, 161
Mending 91, 93, 95
Mercury 34

Metabolic 55, 56, 121, 131
Metabolizing 120
Metal 32, 33, 37
Metals 55
Metastatic 106, 142
Micronutrient 46
Micronutrients 54
Microwave 32, 33
Mind-active 135
Mind-body 16, 63, 134
Mind-inactive 135
Mindful 135, 161
Mineral 46, 47, 54, 131
Misunderstanding 65, 83
Modalities 8, 15, 56, 64
Molasses 46, 130
Molecularly 55
Monosatunsaturated 50
Mortality 7, 20, 86, 150, 152
Mosby's 38
Motility 123, 130
Motivation 66
Mourn 99, 150
Multimineral 54
Multivitamin 54
Music 131, 134, 135, 136, 139
Myeloma 6
Nap 57, 97, 129
Narcotic 46, 129
Nature 18, 64, 65, 83, 96, 113, 162
Naturopathic 7, 10, 46, 117, 131
Naturopathy 16
Nausea 13, 45, 46, 47, 62, 110, 119, 120, 125, 126, 138, 144
Nauseated 62, 126
Negativity 75
Negotiation 151
Nervous 6, 131
Neutropenia 13
Notary 145, 146
Nutrient-dense 46
Nutrients 17, 38, 42, 44, 45, 50, 52, 57, 121
Nutrition 14, 44, 45, 46, 50, 56, 140, 143, 144
Nutritional 20, 44, 45, 46, 47, 120, 122, 128, 143
Nutritionally 143
Nutritionist 131
Off-gas 30
Oil 22, 36, 40, 50, 55, 127
Oils 31, 39, 40, 136
Oncologist 10, 12, 13, 14, 106

Onions 49, 52, 118, 126, 133
Oolong 48, 119, 127
Organ 5, 13, 118
Organic 16, 19, 29, 33, 40, 46, 48, 49, 51, 52, 54, 130
Organically 124
Organisms 7, 24, 29
Osteopathic 16
Overwhelmed 5, 9, 69
Overwhelming 80, 82, 111
Painting 67, 136
Palliative 147
Pancreatic 157
Pans 34
Partners 80, 81, 82
Pastor 154
Pathologist 109
Paths 87, 140
Patience 99
PBA 37
Peace 3, 9, 59, 65, 68, 86, 101, 102, 112, 134, 135, 138, 143, 144, 148, 149, 153, 155, 158
Peaceful 47, 58, 134, 135, 136, 150
Perchlorethelyne 30
Peroxide 32
Pesticides 7, 24, 31, 50
Pharmacist 110
Phytochemicals 119
Plant-based 19, 41
Plastic 31, 32, 33, 37
Plus 123
POA 145, 146
Pollution 7
Polycarbonate 31
Polyphenols 48, 50, 119
Porcelain-coated 34
Postmenopausal 51
Practitioner 63, 117, 118, 131
Praise 57, 113, 134
Pray 2, 64, 102, 107, 113, 115, 116, 134, 144
Prayer 2, 16, 68, 107, 113, 114, 115, 116, 134, 135, 137, 141, 159
Prayers 86, 102, 114
Praying 69, 71, 86, 90, 115, 138
Prevention 20, 118
Pro-biotics 16
Procyanidins 48
Proliferation 119
Protein 19, 42, 47, 49, 131
Proteins 16, 42
Psoriasis 18

Psyllium 46, 53, 123, 124, 129, 130
Radiation 7, 8, 10, 11, 12, 13, 44, 45, 56, 73, 96, 105, 106, 119, 140
Radon 34
Regret 1, 28, 87, 88, 89, 97, 152, 156
Relationships 17, 39, 48, 58, 63, 64, 80, 81, 82, 83, 88, 89, 90, 91, 92, 93, 99, 138, 154, 155
Relaxation 56, 131, 134, 135, 136
Religion 136, 138
Religious 101, 112, 113, 137, 138, 148
Resentment 69
Resins 31
Respiratory 30
Restlessness 73
Resuscitated 145
Resveratrol 52
Rheumatism 119
Sarcoma 5
Sclerosis 18
Scriptures 105
Selenium 42, 54, 119
Self 44, 59, 66, 69, 74
Sepsis 143
Septic 26
Siblings 27, 81, 83
Sleep 56, 73, 89, 92, 97, 121, 134, 162
Sluggish 122
Sodium 129
Soil 25, 26, 162
Spice 118
Spices 47, 49, 133
Spiritual 60, 63, 64, 101, 114, 115, 137, 138, 139, 147, 158
Spirituality 16, 63, 68, 86, 137, 138, 141, 153, 156
Spouses 27, 80, 81, 99, 132
Starch 41
Stomach 47, 53, 62, 118, 121
Stool 53, 122, 123, 129
Strength 45, 101, 110, 141, 143, 158
Strengthen 3, 85, 86
Stress 2, 6, 57, 61, 62, 71, 80, 108, 121, 131, 132, 135, 136, 139, 140, 144
Stressed 69, 153
Stressful 108, 134, 136
Sucrose 41

Sugar 18, 41, 42, 48, 51, 52, 74, 119, 124, 128, 131
Sugars 41
Sulfide 26
Supplements 14, 16, 46, 54, 55, 60, 117, 118, 124, 131
Surrendering 59
Survival 45, 60
Survive 8, 26
Survivor 138
Symptoms 16, 18, 30, 45, 62, 72, 73, 109, 139, 141
Synagogues 101
Syndrome 18, 55, 122
Synthetic 31
System 6, 10, 13, 18, 20, 31, 34, 37, 51, 77, 118, 120, 121, 122, 131
Systemic 13, 18
Tea 22, 46, 48, 53, 119, 123, 127, 128
Terminal 72, 80, 85, 86, 87, 101, 138, 139, 151, 154, 156
Terminally 76
Theories 121
Therapeutic 16
Therapies 10, 15, 16, 18, 21, 60, 120
Therapy 13, 16, 44, 55, 125, 131, 136
Thyroid 34
Tobacco 7
Tocopherols 54
Tocotrienols 54
Toxic 24, 25, 26, 28, 30, 31, 32, 33, 34, 35, 37, 109, 120
Toxicity 13
Toxins 7, 24, 25, 27, 61, 120, 121, 123, 128, 131
Tracheotomy 106
Unsulfured 46, 130
USDA 32
Uterus 109
Vacuuming 30
Virus 36
Viruses 119, 122
Visualization 131, 135
Vitamin 46, 52, 54, 118, 119, 124, 131
Vitamins 16, 54, 119
Vomiting 13, 38, 45, 110, 119, 120, 144
Waheguru 112, 136
Water 7, 16, 24, 25, 26, 27, 29, 37, 38, 39, 47, 53, 54, 57, 97, 120, 122, 123, 124, 125, 126, 127, 128, 129, 130, 131, 132, 135, 162
Water-soluble 121
Weil 19, 54, 123, 160
Wellbeing 71, 77, 89, 106, 154
Wellness 1, 7, 15, 24, 59, 63
Western 2, 10, 12, 15, 60, 61, 64, 106, 141, 142
Wills 146
Wine 22, 48, 52
Withdrawn 81, 85, 152
Woman 74, 77, 79, 90, 114, 115
Women 13, 51, 54, 90, 114, 115, 130
Worship 57
Worshipers 154
Worshiping 86
X-ray 106, 107, 109
Xanthones 120
Yahweh 112
Yoga 16, 136, 139
Zinc 119